Head and Neck Surgery

Editors

BRIAN J. MITCHELL
KYLE TUBBS

SURGICAL CLINICS
OF NORTH AMERICA

www.surgical.theclinics.com

Consulting Editor
RONALD F. MARTIN

April 2022 • Volume 102 • Number 2

ELSEVIER

1600 John F. Kennedy Boulevard • Suite 1800 • Philadelphia, Pennsylvania, 19103-2899

http://www.surgical.theclinics.com

SURGICAL CLINICS OF NORTH AMERICA Volume 102, Number 2
April 2022 ISSN 0039–6109, ISBN-13: 978-0-323-84894-7

Editor: John Vassallo, j.vassallo@elsevier.com
Developmental Editor: Arlene Campos

Surgical Clinics of North America (ISSN 0039–6109) is published bimonthly by Elsevier Inc., 360 Park Avenue South, New York, NY 10010-1710. Months of publication are February, April, June, August, October, and December. Business and Editorial Offices: 1600 John F. Kennedy Blvd., Suite 1800, Philadelphia, PA 19103-2899. Periodicals postage paid at New York, NY and additional mailing offices. Subscription prices are $456.00 per year for US individuals, $1240.00 per year for US institutions, $100.00 per year for US & Canadian students and residents, $547.00 per year for Canadian individuals, $1283.00 per year for Canadian institutions, $552.00 for international individuals, $1283.00 per year for international institutions and $250.00 per year for foreign students/residents. To receive student/resident rate, orders must be accompanied by name of affiliated institution, date of term, and the *signature* of program/residency coordinator on institution letterhead. Orders will be billed at individual rate until proof of status is received. Foreign air speed delivery is included in all *Clinics* subscription prices. All prices are subject to change without notice. POSTMASTER: Send address changes to *Surgical Clinics*, Elsevier Health Sciences Division, Subscription Customer Service, 3251 Riverport Lane, Maryland Heights, MO 63043. **Customer Service (orders, claims, online, change of address): Telephone: 1-800-654-2452 (U.S. and Canada); 314-447-8871 (outside U.S. and Canada). Fax: 314-447-8029. E-mail: journalscustomerservice-usa@elsevier.com (for print support); journalsonlinesupport-usa@elsevier.com (for online support).**

Reprints. For copies of 100 or more, of articles in this publication, please contact the Commercial Reprints Department, Elsevier Inc., 360 Park Avenue South, New York, New York 10010-1710. Tel. 212-633-3874, Fax: 212-633-3820, E-mail: reprints@elsevier.com.

The Surgical Clinics of North America is also published in Spanish by McGraw-Hill Interamericana Editores S.A., P.O. Box 5-237 06500 Mexico D.F. Mexico; and in Portuguese by Interlivros Edicoes Ltda., Rua Comandante Coelho 1085, CEP 21250, Rio de Janeiro, Brazil; and in Greek by Paschalidis Medical Publications, Athens Greece.

The Surgical Clinics of North America is covered in *MEDLINE/PubMed (Index Medicus)*, *EMBASE/Excerpta Medica, Current Contents/Clinical Medicine, Current Contents/Life Sciences, Science Citation Index*, and *ISI/BIOMED*.

Contributors

CONSULTING EDITOR

RONALD F. MARTIN, MD, FACS
Colonel (Retired), United States Army, Department of General Surgery, Pullman Surgical Associates, Pullman Regional Hospital and Clinic Network, Pullman, Washington

EDITORS

BRIAN J. MITCHELL, DO
Otolaryngology–Head and Neck Surgery, Multicare Rockwood Clinic ENT Center, Spokane, Washington

KYLE TUBBS, MD
Otolaryngology, Glacier Ear, Nose, and Throat, Kalispell, Montana

AUTHORS

KELLY G. ANDERSON, MD
Otolaryngologist–Head and Neck Surgeon, Madigan Army Medical Center, Tacoma, Washington

KODY BOLK, MD
Department of Otolaryngology–Head and Neck Surgery, Louisiana State University Health Sciences Center, New Orleans, Louisiana

NEIL N. CHHEDA, MD
Associate Professor, Division of Laryngology, Chief, Residency Program Director, Department of Otolaryngology, University of Florida, Gainesville, Florida

DEREK A. ESCALANTE, MD
Otolaryngologist–Head and Neck Surgeon, Madigan Army Medical Center, Tacoma, Washington

ZACHARY DAVID GUSS, MD, MSc
Deaconess Hospital Radiation Oncology, MultiCare Health System, Spokane, Washington

JEFFREY J. HOULTON, MD
Associate Professor, Otolaryngology–Head and Neck Surgery, University of Washington, Seattle, Washington

JASON P. HUNT, MD, FACS
Division of Otolaryngology, Department of Surgery, University of Utah, Huntsman Cancer Institute, Salt Lake City, Utah

ALBERT L. MERATI, MD
Professor, Chief of the Division of Laryngology, Department of Otolaryngology–Head and Neck Surgery, University of Washington, Seattle, Washington

TANYA K. MEYER, MD
Associate Professor in Laryngology, Residency Program Director, Department of Otolaryngology–Head and Neck Surgery, University of Washington, Seattle, Washington

KURT MUELLER, MD
Department of Otolaryngology–Head and Neck Surgery, Louisiana State University Health Sciences Center, New, Orleans, Louisiana

CASSIE PAN, MD
Resident Physician, Department of Otolaryngology–Head and Neck Surgery, University of Washington, Washington

JOHN PANG, MD
Fellow in Head and Neck Oncology and Microvascular Reconstruction, University of Washington, Seattle, Washington

NEELAM PHALKE, MD
Department of Otolaryngology–Head and Neck Surgery, Louisiana State University Health Sciences Center, New, Orleans, Louisiana

ZAIN RIZVI, MD
Assistant Professor, Department of Otolaryngology–Head and Neck Surgery, University of Washington, Seattle, Washington

JORDAN P. SAND, MD, FACS
Sand Plastic Surgery, Spokane, Washington; University of Washington School of Medicine, Seattle, Washington; Washington State University School of Medicine

LAUREN SLATTERY, MD
Department of Surgery, University of Utah, Salt Lake City, Utah

ROHAN R. WALVEKAR, MD
Department of Otolaryngology–Head and Neck Surgery, Louisiana State University Health Sciences Center, New, Orleans, Louisiana

GRACE M. WANDELL, MD, MS
Resident, Department of Otolaryngology–Head and Neck Surgery, University of Washington, Seattle, Washington

Contents

Esophageal dysphagia presents acutely, most frequently as a food impaction, or in a progressive fashion. Anatomic changes are frequently responsible. Although the history may be suggestive, diagnosis is made from imaging or endoscopic studies. In asymptomatic cases, observation is most appropriate. Treatment is frequently accomplished endoscopically. Strictures, cricopharyngeal hyperfunction, and Zenker diverticulum are potential etiologic causes. For the purpose of this article focused on upper esophageal dysphagia, delineation between the upper and lower parts is the crossing of the aortic arch but also includes the most distal aspects of the hypopharynx including the inferior pharyngeal constrictors and upper esophageal sphincter.

 Video content accompanies this article at http://www.surgical. theclinics.com

In this section, we discuss the management of benign salivary gland disease. Pathologies vary from sialolithiasis, salivary duct stenosis, sialadenitis, infectious glandular disease, autoimmune glandular disease, and radioactive iodine-induced disease. We discuss both novel techniques in the diagnosis and management of these diseases, including ultrasound, sialendoscopy, minor salivary gland biopsy, and botulinum toxin injection, which allow for both the alleviation of symptoms and gland preservation.

The online physician image is a point of emerging importance in the field of medicine. Online information has become critically important to patients who are seeking out care. Leaving online reviews has become a common practice among patients and as such, physician practices have embraced the use of social media to help grow their online presence. In addition, attention to online review sites has come to be an important part of protecting a physician's image. This article will discuss the importance of engaging the physician online review sites and help identify strategies for reviewing and improving a physician's online image.

Oral cavity cancer represents a heterogeneous group of cancers with unique etiologic, diagnostic, and treatment considerations based on the subsite. While decreases in smoking have resulted in the development of fewer oral cavity cancers, the incidence remains high in certain geographic areas. History and physical examination, as well as tissue biopsy, are key to diagnosis. Although surgical resection is the primary treatment modality for oral cavity cancer, the optimal treatment plan for a patient is an individualized approach accounting for comorbidities, goals of care, and functional outcomes related to speech and swallowing.

Salivary cancers are rare tumors that arise in major and minor salivary glands. Workup almost always includes fine-needle aspiration or core needle biopsy in select cases. Imaging with ultrasound, computed tomography, or MRI is also helpful, particularly with MRI to assess facial nerve involvement or skull base involvement. Preserving function of the facial nerve is of paramount importance, and the standard of care is to not sacrifice facial nerve except in instances of gross encasement and inability to dissect tumor off of the nerve. Adjuvant radiation and chemotherapy offer survival advantages for select patients.

SURGICAL CLINICS
OF NORTH AMERICA

SERIES OF RELATED INTEREST

Advances in Surgery
https://www.advancessurgery.com/
Surgical Oncology Clinics
https://www.surgonc.theclinics.com/
Thoracic Surgery Clinics
http://www.thoracic.theclinics.com/

THE CLINICS ARE AVAILABLE ONLINE!
Access your subscription at:
www.theclinics.com

Foreword
Head and Neck Surgery

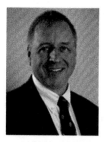

Ronald F. Martin, MD, FACS
Consulting Editor

Readers of *Surgical Clinics* for any length of time are familiar that a great many of our issues cover topics that span clinical areas with specialty and subspecialty overlap. This issue, guest edited by our colleagues Drs Tubbs and Mitchell, on surgery of the Head and Neck is one of the best examples of that overlap. On one level, it makes perfect sense that specialist care for surgery of the Head and Neck has rapidly solidified its hold on the aspects of care while other disorders are cared for by a broader range of clinicians. Improvements in imaging and less-invasive clinical therapeutic options have helped to secure the need for significant consolidation of specialty and subspecialty care for many maladies of the head and neck. On another level, resource availability, provider distribution, and geographic disparities in resources yield an imperative that some of this care capability should remain in the hands of the more generalist clinician.

Historically, these opposing forces have been sources for internecine disputes that have played out in multiple fora. While some of that may still exist, tension along those lines may be reducing. There are many possible explanations for this. A moderate- to longer-term evaluation may suggest that specialization and hyperspecialization have gained greater acceptance among patients and physicians alike: reducing the basis for "turf war"–type concerns. Individual providers, even in rural or austere settings, have chosen to "pick their battles" (if you will) on just how much clinical ground to hold on to and how much to refer away. An analysis viewed through the prism of more recent events might also include that referral patterns are altered by the effects of the pandemic, in particular, with its impact on personnel, capacity, and equipment resources.

From the altitudinal viewpoint, the major forces that will shape how we best flow our patients and care from one environment to another are most likely to be business related. Consolidations of smaller health care entities into larger ones, better defined business agreements between systems that share geographic and regional interests, and the ever-increasing percentage of physicians who are employed by larger entities

Surg Clin N Am 102 (2022) ix–x
https://doi.org/10.1016/j.suc.2022.02.002
0039-6109/22/© 2022 Published by Elsevier Inc.

surgical.theclinics.com

will reshape the resource availability, distribution, and incentives that ultimately decide where patients receive their care and from whom. Also, our continued ability to provide much care—even complex care—on an outpatient or near-outpatient basis will favor consolidation of care into entities that provide complex care without requiring acute care hospital level resources. These smaller, more focused enterprises will likely benefit from improved fiscal agility compared with larger competitors, who must factor in costly reserves in staffing and resources for a broader spectrum of concerns.

As with so many other topics, the view from altitude and the view from the ground are related but dissimilar. We, as stewards of care for our patients and our communities, must maintain broad knowledge and detailed knowledge to be effective in our roles. Administratively, we must be cognizant of the gains and losses to smaller and larger organizations as we siphon off care from one environment to another. Loss of situational awareness of the systemic fragility this can add imperils both the care-providing enterprises and the patient community as well in times of stress.

Our relationships between and among generalists and specialists have similar concerns. From a clinical standpoint, it benefits general surgeons (whether they work in larger or smaller enterprises) to have an excellent understanding of the knowledge and capabilities of our Head and Neck colleagues. Whether we are to care for a patient on a more local basis or whether referrals need to be made to those with more extensive specialty knowledge, a sound basis for understanding and communication can only help. We are indebted to Drs Tubbs and Mitchell, along with their colleagues, for providing us with the excellent collection of articles to help us have a better knowledge base.

On the macro level, we physicians need to have an excellent and deep understanding of resource capability and distribution. Even if an individual does not work in the administrative arena, clinician input is necessary and vital for our administrative partners to make decisions that truly improve the provision of care to our communities and not just address more restrictive financial concerns. At the *Surgical Clinics*, we strive to bring the readership content in context to help us all better serve our patients and improve our capabilities. We are grateful for those who contribute to the series and very grateful to the readership for their support and feedback. Stay safe and be well.

Ronald F. Martin, MD, FACS
Colonel (retired), United States Army Reserve
Department of General Surgery
Pullman Surgical Associates
Pullman Regional Hospital and Clinic Network
825 Southeast Bishop Boulevard, Suite 130
Pullman, WA 99163, USA

E-mail address:
rfmcescna@gmail.com

Preface

Head and Neck Surgery

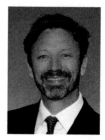 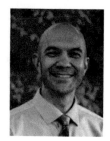

Brian J. Mitchell, DO   Kyle Tubbs, MD
Editors

We are excited to bring you this issue of *Surgical Clinics* focusing on head and neck surgery. As any surgeon knows, the head and neck region is filled with fascinating, complex anatomy. During cadaveric dissection, medical students marvel at the shear amount of critical structures contained in this relatively small area of the body, and nearly every surgical procedure in the head and neck involves dissection around one of these critical structures. Both General Surgeons and Otolaryngologists spend time working in the head and neck as they address benign and malignant neoplasms, endocrine problems, traumatic injuries, and speech/swallowing disorders. Both General Surgeons and Otolaryngologists will see patients in clinic with head and neck complaints.

This issue of *Surgical Clinics* contains articles discussing head and neck cancer management as well as workup and treatment of head and neck functional problems (dysphagia and salivary gland dysfunction). There are also articles focusing on appropriate management of thyroid and parathyroid disease. The upper airway is the most critical structure contained within the neck and receives special attention in this issue.

As an added bonus, we are also happy to present an article pertaining to physician reputation in the era of frequent on-line reviews and social media posts. This topic is only increasing in relevance, and nearly every practitioner is affected by it. While we often cannot control what someone "posts" about our care, it is critical to be aware of the tools available to us to protect our practice and reputation.

Most of us in the field of Otolaryngology selected the specialty because we were enthralled with the anatomic detail in the head and neck. We know many General

Surg Clin N Am 102 (2022) xi–xii
https://doi.org/10.1016/j.suc.2022.02.001
0039-6109/22/© 2022 Published by Elsevier Inc.
surgical.theclinics.com

Surgeons feel the same way. We hope this issue will prove useful to physicians in training as well as physicians in practice, as they approach head and neck diseases.

Brian J. Mitchell, DO
Otolaryngology/Head & Neck Surgery
Multicare Rockwood Clinic ENT Center
Spokane, WA 99204, USA

Kyle Tubbs, MD
Otolaryngology
Glacier Ear, Nose, and Throat
Kalispell MT 59901, USA

E-mail addresses:
nwnecksurgeon@gmail.com (B.J. Mitchell)
tubbskyle@yahoo.com (K. Tubbs)

Upper Esophageal Dysphagia

Neil N. Chheda, MD

KEYWORDS

- Esophageal dysphagia • Stricture • Cricopharyngeal hyperfunction
- Zenker diverticulum

KEY POINTS

- When symptomatic, esophageal dysphagia most frequently presents with solid dysphagia.
- Endoscopic technique may result in symptom improvement.
- The cricopharyngeus muscle is at the junction of the pharynx and esophagus and plays a key role in upper esophageal sphincter dysfunction and Zenker diverticulum formation.

INTRODUCTION

The esophageal phase is the third and final part of the swallow process. Like the second pharyngeal phase, it is under involuntary control. Its purpose is to transport the food bolus prepared during the first oral phase from the pharynx to the stomach to continue the rest of the digestive process. Normal esophageal transit times range from 5 to 10 seconds for nectar and pudding-thick food consistencies, depending on body position.[1] In addition to the intrinsic features of the esophagus, the esophageal phase is affected by the preceding pharyngeal phase, the successive gastric anatomy and physiology, extrinsic cervical and thoracic anatomic structures, and systemic diseases.

Although a continuous structure, differences exist between the upper and the lower parts of the esophagus. Skeletal muscle dominates the upper portion, whereas smooth muscle is the dominant form found in the lower esophagus. For the purpose of this article focused on upper esophageal dysphagia, the delineation between the upper and lower parts is the crossing of the aortic arch but also includes the most distal aspects of the hypopharynx including the inferior pharyngeal constrictors and upper esophageal sphincter (UES). Because most esophageal dysmotility occurs in the smooth muscle portion, esophageal motility disorders are beyond the scope of this article.[2]

Division of Laryngology, Department of Otolaryngology, University of Florida, 1345 Center Drive, PO Box 100264, Gainesville, FL 32610, USA
E-mail address: neil.chheda@ent.ufl.edu

Surg Clin N Am 102 (2022) 199–207
https://doi.org/10.1016/j.suc.2021.12.002
0039-6109/22/© 2022 Elsevier Inc. All rights reserved.

HISTORY

Common upper esophageal dysphagia symptoms include solid and pill dysphagia, odynophagia, regurgitation of undigested food, chest or abdominal pain, weight loss, and aspiration with associated pneumonia. Dysphagia to liquids tends to be a later symptom. Symptoms are frequently progressive with an acute onset suggestive of an obstruction, such as a food impaction event. Relevant past medical history includes systemic inflammatory diseases, reflux, trauma, and radiation history to the head and neck region or thoracic cavity. Hemoptysis may be a more ominous sign of a malignancy.

PHYSICAL EXAMINATION

The physical examination tends to be nonspecific. A wet "gurgly" voice may be suggestive of pharyngeal residue caused by incomplete clearance of saliva and food bolus from an impaired esophageal phase. The physical examination may, however, provide insights into the potential for interventions. Limitations of neck flexion and extension, cervical kyphosis, trismus, and the presence of mandibular tori can affect the feasibility of transoral interventions.

LABORATORY AND RADIOLOGY

Laboratory analysis does not play a large role in the work-up of upper esophageal dysphagia. Radiographic studies, particularly fluoroscopy, are frequently used in the analysis of solid food dysphagia. Barium swallow studies have been found to be near 95% sensitive for cervical esophageal narrowing.[3] A water-soluble contrast, instead of barium, may be considered in cases of suspected perforation or leak to decrease mediastinal reaction. Endoscopy may be used for diagnosis, intervention, or to evaluate for malignancy. However, endoscopy may underrecognize luminal narrowing. Esophagoscopy is diagnostic and therapeutic and may take the form of rigid transoral, flexible transoral, and flexible transnasal. A relative advantage of the transnasal approach is the ability to perform without the need for sedation. Interventions may be coupled to diagnostic endoscopic procedures. Malignancies that may present with lumen narrowing most commonly include primary esophageal adenocarcinoma and squamous cell carcinoma. Less frequently, metastatic lesions may present in the esophagus. In cases of malignancy, thoracic computed tomography and endoscopic ultrasound evaluation may be indicated. Reflux and motility may be assessed through pH probes including capsule and catheter-based systems; impedance; manometry; or radiographic studies, such as scintigraphy.[4]

FOOD IMPACTION

Esophageal food impaction may present as an acute dysphagia scenario. Food impaction is the third most common nonbiliary gastroenterology emergency seen, after upper and lower gastrointestinal bleeds.[5] Patients with food impactions frequently have underlying esophageal pathology including esophagitis, strictures, hiatal hernia, or other obstructing masses with estimates of an abnormality found in nearly 80% of impaction cases. Approximately 20% of food impactions occur in the upper esophagus. For food material, the offending obstruction may be endoscopically "pulled out" or "pushed" into the stomach. Although less effective in those with underlying structural abnormalities, glucagon may be considered to relax the smooth muscles of the esophagus to aid in the successful distal passage of the food bolus.[6]

BENIGN NARROWING OF THE ESOPHAGUS

Benign strictures may present anywhere in the upper esophagus. Although mild narrowing may be asymptomatic, with greater compromise of luminal patency patients may present with solid food or pill dysphagia. Compromise of the lumen of greater than 50% tends to cause symptoms.[7] Other esophageal symptoms may include regurgitation, chest pain, and abdominal pain.

There are multiple causes for benign esophageal strictures. Although reflux-related Schatzki rings occur in the lower esophagus near the gastroesophageal junction, gastroesophageal reflux–related narrowing may also occur in the upper esophagus. Some of these strictures may be related to an ectopic gastric mucosa patch.[8] Inflammatory conditions of the esophagus that may be associated with stricture formation include eosinophilic esophagitis and lymphocytic esophagitis.[9] Other associated systemic diseases include scleroderma, epidermolysis bullosa, and pemphigus.[10]

Trauma and iatrogenic origins may also result in stricture formation. Caustic ingestion after accidental or suicidal ingestion may result in scarring, fibrosis, and esophageal narrowing.[11] Stricture formation may occur after the resection and reconstructive anastomosis in the surgical treatment of malignancies of the esophagus and head and neck region. Even in the absence of surgical treatment, radiation therapy alone of the head and neck or thoracic region may result in stricture formation. Postradiation stricture formation more frequently occurs during the late phase of treatment.[12]

Esophageal webs are thin extensions of the esophageal mucosa that may obstruct the lumen. Plummer-Vinson syndrome, a rare disorder, presents with the triad of dysphagia, iron deficiency anemia, and an upper esophageal web.[13] Those with Plummer-Vinson syndrome have a higher risk of developing hypopharyngeal squamous cell carcinoma.

Because not all strictures are symptomatic, observation may be indicated for those that do not significantly impact the lumen. Dilation is often the first-line treatment, when needed. Various types of esophageal bougie or push dilators are available. A Maloney dilator is a tapered, weighted bougie used without a guidewire. The Savary-Gillard system (Cook Medical, Bloomington, IN) is also tapered but are designed to be used with a guidewire. Nontapered Hurst type and metallic wire guided Eders are less commonly used.[14] Balloon dilation may also be performed for the dilation of upper esophageal strictures without the theoretic shearing, longitudinal forces seen with bougie dilation.[15] A meta-analysis found no difference between complications, perforation rate, symptom relief, and recurrence when comparing bougie versus balloon dilating devices.[16]

Dilations may be safely performed under general anesthesia, with sedation or in an unsedated fashion.[17] Advantages of unsedated procedures include reducing the risk of anesthesia complications. A 2007 national survey of endoscopists found that unplanned cardiopulmonary events secondary to conscious sedation constitute most endoscopy complications because 67% of complications and 72% of mortalities were cardiopulmonary related.[18] Fluoroscopy is used as an adjuvant tool particularly in complex strictures or with severe narrowing where the distal side cannot be visualized. Complications associated with dilation include esophageal perforation, bleeding, and anesthesia complications.

Recurrence of the narrowing after dilation is not uncommon. Antireflux and antiacid treatment may be considered with agents, such as proton pump inhibitors and histamine-2 receptor antagonists. Other adjuvant treatments include intralesional steroid injection and the use of topical mitomycin C.[19] Stent placement may be indicated in cases of malignancy or fistula. However, stents may migrate or cause further erosion and are not considered first-line treatment.[20] Case series of patients performing self-dilations have been published since the 1980s and have shown patient satisfaction, efficacy, and safety.[21]

Strictures with complete or near complete obliteration of the lumen may not be amenable to traditional anterograde dilation. A combined anterograde and retrograde technique referred to as a rendezvous may be performed using peroral anterograde approach and retrograde visualization through a gastrotomy site.[22] In severe cases, such as after caustic ingestion, esophagectomy with colonic interposition or gastric pull up or esophageal bypass may be considered.[23]

Although not causing a true reduction in lumen size, external compression of the esophagus may cause a functional decrease in luminal size thereby producing similar symptoms. An aberrant right subclavian artery, or double or right-sided aortic arch may cause a posterior compression of the esophageal because of its posterior course to the esophagus resulting in the process known as dysphagia lusoria.[24] Left-sided heart enlargement and aortic enlargement may also impose on the esophagus.[25] Masses, particularly of the mediastinum, may also cause an external compression and include such entities as thyroid, thymus, and mediastinal adenopathy. Cervical spine osteophytes as may be seen in diffuse idiopathic skeletal hyperostosis can also cause compression.[26]

DYSFUNCTION OF THE UPPER ESOPHAGEAL SPHINCTER

The UES is situated at the junction of the pharyngeal and esophageal phases of swallow. It is comprised of the pharyngeal inferior constrictor muscles, the cricopharyngeus, and the upper esophageal muscles.[27] It rests in a contracted state thereby preventing excessive air swallowing and esophagopharyngeal reflux. During the normal swallow process, the UES opens in a five-step process:

1) Inhibition of the tonic contraction
2) Elevation of the hyoid-laryngeal complex, which results in passive opening
3) Passage of the food bolus, which distends the UES
4) Subsequent collapse of the UES when the bolus passes through
5) Active contraction, which leads to closure of the UES

Dysfunction of the UES, also known as cricopharyngeal (CP) hyperfunction, CP dysfunction, or CP achalasia, may result in dysphagia, globus, odynophagia, regurgitation, or a choking sensation. The failure of the cricopharyngeus to relax and open causes an obstruction to bolus transfer. Diagnosis is seen on fluoroscopic examination with a "CP bar" being seen as a posterior impression on the esophagus, usually at the level of C5 or C6.[28] Quantitative data are seen on manometry, which may also identify lower esophageal dysfunction or esophageal body dysmotility.[29] Laryngoscopy examination may give indirect signs of UES dysfunction including preswallow pooling of secretions, postswallow hypopharyngeal residue, or regurgitation into the pyriform sinuses.[30]

Dysfunction may be caused by functional or structural reasons. Functional CP dysfunction refers to the failure of UES relaxation and has been associated with brainstem infarction, high vagal injury, traumatic brain injury, and other neurologic degenerative diseases.[31] Structural CP dysfunction also results in improper opening of the UES despite relaxation of the UES musculature. Structural CP dysfunction is commonly found in postradiation patients.[32] Failure of the UES to relax may also occur in the setting of esophageal dysmotility, gastroesophageal reflux disease, or be idiopathic.

Particularly in structural CP, as may be seen after the treatment of patients with head and neck cancer, dilation may be considered as a first-line treatment. Much like for a benign stricture, dilation is conducted by similar devices and under varied levels of sedation, including unsedated.[33] Recurrence of symptoms after dilation is not uncommon.

Botulism toxin (BTX) injections have been found to be effective for the treatment of the failure to relax, achalasia, of the cricopharyngeus with success rates of swallow improvement ranging from 43% to 100%.[34] Effectiveness depends on the dosage used and cause of the dysfunction. BTX injections may be performed in conjunction with dilation when performed endoscopically. Localization during percutaneous approaches may be done with use of electromyography or image guidance with computed tomography or fluoroscopy.[35] Complications associated with BTX injections include worsening of swallow, belching, esophagopharyngeal reflux, and vocal fold movement impairment. Given the pharmacologic properties of BTX, these complications are most frequently temporary. Those who respond well to BTX but have recurrence of symptoms, may later be candidates for CP myotomy (**Fig. 1**).

Myotomy of the cricopharyngeus may offer longer symptom improvement than dilation or BTX injection in the appropriate patient population. Myotomy may be done via a transcervical approach under general or sedation anesthesia. Myotomy should extend superiorly and include a portion of the inferior pharyngeal constrictors and inferiorly to include a portion of the upper esophageal musculature.

An endoscopic approach to the cricopharyngeus has also been described as a safe alternative to open surgery.[36] The endoscopic myotomy is frequently accomplished with use of a carbon dioxide laser. Similar to an open approach, myotomy is extended into the inferior pharyngeal constrictors and upper esophageal fibers. The depth of the myotomy is the buccopharyngeal fascia. Entry into the deeper retropharyngeal space or alar fascia significantly increases the risk of mediastinitis.

PHARYNGEAL AND UPPER ESOPHAGEAL DIVERTICULUM

Zenker diverticulum (ZD) are the most frequently diverticulum that occur in the upper esophageal region. They are most frequent in the older population. ZD are a pulsion-

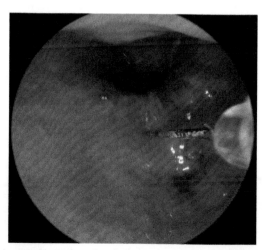

Fig. 1. A needle is inserted into the cricopharyngeus muscle under direct endoscopic visualization. Mild abrasions are noted of the esophageal introitus after dilation.

false diverticulum that occur between the inferior pharyngeal constrictors and the cricopharyngeus. This region of relative weakness is referred to as Killian triangle.[37] The common wall between the diverticulum and the esophagus is the cricopharyngeus. Because it is a false diverticulum, the muscle is not involved and only the mucosa and submucosal layers are contained in the sac. CP hyperfunction is noted in almost all cases of ZD. One hypothesis for the formation of the diverticulum is the increased pharyngeal pressure needed during swallow to overcome the higher CP pressures causes a herniation of the submucosal and mucosal layers through Killian triangle. Prevalence ranges from 0.01% to 0.11% of the population but this may underestimate those with asymptomatic or minimally symptomatic dysphagia. Symptoms include regurgitation of chewed but not digested food, halitosis, cough, and aspiration. Diagnosis may be made from fluoroscopic study or endoscopy. Fluoroscopy is used to confirm the origin of the diverticulum superior to the cricopharyngeus differentiating it from other rarer diverticulum types.

Treatment may include observation for nonsymptomatic pouches, open techniques, and endoscopic techniques. Almost all of the techniques involve a CP myotomy. Open techniques include a CP myotomy alone, diverticulopexy, and diverticulectomy with or without myotomy. Endoscopic techniques can include rigid and flexible options. Rigid technique involves visualization of the ZD and the esophagus with division of the common wall, most frequently with stapling device (**Fig. 2**).[38] Use of the carbon dioxide laser and harmonic scalpel have also been safely performed. Limitations to rigid technique include cervical anatomy and jaw opening size, which may prevent proper visualization. To overcome visualization limitations, flexible technique has been described using argon cautery, hook knife, or bipolar or monopolar forceps.[39]

Occurring less frequently, non-ZD of the upper esophagus may also present with dysphagia. Although also a false, pulsion-type diverticulum like a ZD, a Killian-Jamieson diverticulum herniates inferior to the cricopharyngeus and the superolateral esophageal fibers and presents more anteriorly than a ZD. Because of proximity to the recurrent laryngeal nerve, open resection is recommended, although endoscopic interventions have also been safely described.[40] Because it originates inferior to the CP, the role of myotomy is unclear. Laimer diverticulum are even more uncommon with less than five described in the medical literature. Like a Killian-Jamieson

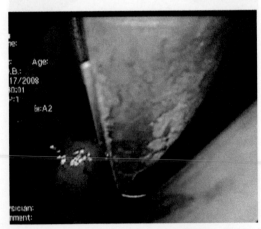

Fig. 2. A stapler device is seen around the common wall between the anterior esophagus and posterior Zenker diverticulum.

diverticulum, they originate inferior to the CP but instead are directed more posteriorly through the Laimer-Haeckerman triangle. Open surgery has been described without need for myotomy.

Traction diverticulum may present from inflammation of the mediastinum or from cervical spine hardware.[41] In cases associated with spinal hardware inflammation, open surgery may be considered if intervention is warranted because this can also address the underlying cervical plate at the same time.

SUMMARY

Esophageal dysphagia most frequently presents as solid dysphagia. Diagnosis is made by imaging or endoscopy. Endoscopic interventions are effective, although recurrence of symptoms is not uncommon.

CLINICS CARE POINTS

- When evaluating a patient with a symptomatic upper esophageal stricture, consider the degree of trismus and neck anatomic restrictions, which may preclude a per-oral approach.
- When evaluating a patient with suspected cricopharyngeal dysfunction, evaluate for potential cause and esophageal function. Attempts to reduce cricopharyngeal hyperfunction in the setting of esophageal dysmotility may result in esophagopharyngeal reflux.
- When evaluating a patient with suspected diverticulum, evaluate the relationship of the diverticulum to the cricopharyngeus. A Zenker diverticulum originates superior to the cricopharyngeus. Other types of diverticulum, such as a Killian-Jamieson, originate inferior to the cricopharyngeus. Although a Zenker diverticulum is safely treated endoscopically, this per oral approach may result in injury to the recurrent laryngeal nerve if used for other types of diverticulum.

DISCLOSURE

The author has nothing to disclose.

REFERENCES

1. Garand KLF, Culp L, Wang B, et al. Aging effects on esophageal transit time in the upright position during video fluoroscopy. Ann Otol Rhinol Laryngol 2020; 129(6):618–24.
2. Gyawali CP, Sifrim D, Carlson DA, et al. Ineffective esophageal motility: concepts, future directions, and conclusions from the Stanford 2018 symposium. Neurogastroenterol Motil 2019;31(9):e13584.
3. West J, Kim CH, Reichert Z, et al. Esophagram findings in cervical esophageal stenosis: a case-controlled quantitative analysis. Laryngoscope 2018;128(9): 2022–8.
4. Vardar R, Keskin M. Indications of 24-h esophageal pH monitoring, capsule pH monitoring, combined pH monitoring with multichannel impedance, esophageal manometry, radiology and scintigraphy in gastroesophageal reflux disease? Turk J Gastroenterol 2017;28(Suppl 1):S16–21.
5. Gurala D, Polavarapu A, Philipose J, et al. Esophageal food impaction: a retrospective chart review. Gastroenterol Res 2021;14(3):173–8.

6. Alaradi O, Bartholomew M, Barkin JS. Upper endoscopy and glucagon: a new technique in the management of acute esophageal food impaction. Am J Gastroenterol 2001;96(3):912–3.

7. Adler DG, Siddiqui AA. Endoscopic management of esophageal strictures. Gastrointest Endosc 2017;86(1):35–43.

8. Chong VH. Clinical significance of heterotopic gastric mucosal patch of the proximal esophagus. World J Gastroenterol 2013;19(3):331–8.

9. Navarro P, Laserna-Mendieta EJ, Guagnozzi D, et al, EUREOS EoE CONNECT research group. Proton pump inhibitor therapy reverses endoscopic features of fibrosis in eosinophilic esophagitis. Dig Liver Dis 2021;53(11):1479–85.

10. Boregowda U, Goyal H, Mann R, et al. Endoscopic management of benign recalcitrant esophageal strictures. Ann Gastroenterol 2021;34(3):287–99.

11. Hall AH, Jacquemin D, Henny D, et al. Corrosive substances ingestion: a review. Crit Rev Toxicol 2019;49(8):637–69.

12. Francis DO, Hall E, Dang JH, et al. Outcomes of serial dilation for high-grade radiation-related esophageal strictures in head and neck cancer patients. Laryngoscope 2015;125(4):856–62.

13. Petrea OC, Stanciu C, Muzica CM, et al. Idiopathic cervical esophageal webs: a case report and literature review. Int J Gen Med 2020;13:1123–7.

14. Khanna N. How do I dilate a benign esophageal stricture? Can J Gastroenterol 2006;20(3):153–5.

15. Maejima R, Iijima K, Koike T, et al. Endoscopic balloon dilatation for pharyngoupper esophageal stricture after treatment of head and neck cancer. Dig Endosc 2015;27(3):310–6.

16. Josino IR, Madruga-Neto AC, Ribeiro IB, et al. Endoscopic dilation with bougies versus balloon dilation in esophageal benign strictures: systematic review and meta-analysis. Gastroenterol Res Pract 2018;2018:5874870.

17. Lerner MZ, Bourdillon AT, Dai F, et al. Safety considerations for esophageal dilation by anesthetic type: a systematic review. Am J Otol 2021;42(5):103128.

18. Sharma VK, Nguyen CC, Crowell MD, et al. A national study of cardiopulmonary unplanned events after GI endoscopy. Gastrointest Endosc 2007;66:27–34.

19. Méndez-Nieto CM, Zarate-Mondragón F, Ramírez-Mayans J, et al. Topical mitomycin C versus intralesional triamcinolone in the management of esophageal stricture due to caustic ingestion. Rev Gastroenterol Mex 2015;80(4):248–54.

20. Godin A, Liberman M. The modern approach to esophageal palliative and emergency surgery. Ann Transl Med 2021;9(10):905.

21. Alwan M, Giddings CE. Self-dilatation of benign oesophageal strictures: a literature review. ANZ J Surg 2021. https://doi.org/10.1111/ans.16775.

22. Liu D, Pickering T, Kokot N, et al. Outcomes of combined antegrade-retrograde dilations for radiation-induced esophageal strictures in head and neck cancer patients. Dysphagia 2021. https://doi.org/10.1007/s00455-020-10236-6.

23. Tustumi F, Seguro FCBDC, Szachnowicz S, et al. Surgical management of esophageal stenosis due to ingestion of corrosive substances. J Surg Res 2021;264:249–59.

24. Wellington J, Kim J, Castell DO, et al. Dysphagia lusoria: utility of high-resolution impedance manometry to identify true disease. Neurogastroenterol Motil 2021;e14176.

25. Massaro N, Verro B, Greco G, et al. Dyspnea in patient with arteria lusoria: a case report. Iran J Otorhinolaryngol 2020;32(112):333–6.

26. Scholz C, Naseri Y, Hohenhaus M, et al. Long-term results after surgical treatment of diffuse idiopathic skeletal hyperostosis (DISH) causing dysphagia. J Clin Neurosci 2019;67:151–5.
27. Kahrilas PJ, Dodds WJ, Dent J, et al. Upper esophageal sphincter function during deglutition. Gastroenterology 1988;95(1):52–62.
28. Dewan K, Santa Maria C, Noel J. Cricopharyngeal achalasia: management and associated outcomes: a scoping review. Otolaryngol Head Neck Surg 2020; 163(6):1109–13.
29. Blais P, Bennett MC, Gyawali CP. Upper esophageal sphincter metrics on high-resolution manometry differentiate etiologies of esophagogastric junction outflow obstruction. Neurogastroenterol Motil 2019;31(5):e13558.
30. Weiland DJ, Goshtasbi K, Verma SP. Fiberoptic endoscopic evaluation of swallowing findings in individuals with Zenker's diverticulum and cricopharyngeal bar. Eur Arch Otorhinolaryngol 2020;277(7):2017–21.
31. Gilheaney Ó, Kerr P, Béchet S, et al. Effectiveness of endoscopic cricopharyngeal myotomy in adults with neurological disease: systematic review. J Laryngol Otol 2016;130(12):1077–85.
32. Dawe N, Patterson J, Hamilton D, et al. Targeted use of endoscopic CO2 laser cricopharyngeal myotomy for improving swallowing function following head and neck cancer treatment. J Laryngol Otol 2014;128(12):1105–10.
33. Dou Z, Zu Y, Wen H, et al. The effect of different catheter balloon dilatation modes on cricopharyngeal dysfunction in patients with dysphagia. Dysphagia 2012; 27(4):514–20.
34. Xie M, Dou Z, Wan G, et al. Design and implementation of botulinum toxin on cricopharyngeal dysfunction guided by a combination of catheter balloon, ultrasound, and electromyography (BECURE) in patients with stroke: study protocol for a randomized, double-blinded, placebo-controlled trial. Trials 2021;22(1):238.
35. Kelly EA, Koszewski IJ, Jaradeh SS, et al. Botulinum toxin injection for the treatment of upper esophageal sphincter dysfunction. Ann Otol Rhinol Laryngol 2013; 122(2):100–8.
36. Pitman M, Weissbrod P. Endoscopic CO2 laser cricopharyngeal myotomy. Laryngoscope 2009;119(1):45–53.
37. Little RE, Bock JM. Pharyngoesophageal diverticuli: diagnosis, incidence and management. Curr Opin Otolaryngol Head Neck Surg 2016;24(6):500–4.
38. Richtsmeier WJ. Endoscopic management of Zenker diverticulum: the staple-assisted approach. Am J Med 2003;(115 Suppl 3A):175S–8S.
39. Beard K, Swanström LL. Zenker's diverticulum: flexible versus rigid repair. J Thorac Dis 2017;9(Suppl 2):S154–62.
40. Saisho K, Matono S, Tanaka T, et al. Surgery for Killian-Jamieson diverticulum: a report of two cases. Surg Case Rep 2020;6:17.
41. Allis TJ, Grant NN, Davidson BJ. Hypopharyngeal diverticulum formation following anterior discectomy and fusion: case series. Ear Nose Throat J 2010; 89(11):E4–9.

Management of Benign Salivary Gland Conditions

Kody Bolk, MD, Kurt Mueller, MD, Neelam Phalke, MD, Rohan R. Walvekar, MD*

KEYWORDS

- Sialolithiasis • Salivary duct stenosis • Sialadenitis • Autoimmune salivary disease

KEY POINTS

- Sialolithiasis is one of the most common causes of sialadenitis. When conservative measures fail, sialendoscopy plays a significant role in endoscopic stone removal or visualization for assistance with a combined transoral approach.
- When working up patients with sialadenitis, it is important to include less common infectious etiologies on the differential diagnosis including HIV, cat-scratch disease, mycobacterial infection, and mumps.
- Minor salivary gland biopsy and sialendoscopy have played increasingly important roles in the diagnosis and management of patients with autoimmune salivary gland disease.
- Sialendoscopy with steroid irrigation, obturator dilation, or stent placement aids in the treatment of salivary duct stenosis and radioactive iodine-induced sialadenitis.

 Video content accompanies this article at http://www.surgical.theclinics.com

INTRODUCTION

Historically, disease of the salivary glands has been classified into neoplastic and non-neoplastic etiologies. Most nonneoplastic etiologies of salivary gland disease stem from chronic inflammatory processes, the management of which has largely been unchanged over several decades. Management commonly includes both medical and surgical intervention. Oftentimes, when medical therapy fails, surgical intervention consists of the removal of the affected glands. However, there has recently been an increase in momentum toward surgical management of these conditions with an emphasis on gland preservation. In this article, we aim to review many of the benign salivary gland disorders, with a focus on the areas of management where an improved understanding of the various disease processes and pathology has created a paradigm shift in management.

Department of Otolaryngology Head & Neck Surgery, Louisiana State University Health Sciences Center, 533 Bolivar Street, Suite 566 New, Orleans, LA 70112, USA
* Corresponding author.
E-mail address: rwalve@lsuhsc.edu

Surg Clin N Am 102 (2022) 209–231
https://doi.org/10.1016/j.suc.2022.01.001
0039-6109/22/© 2022 Elsevier Inc. All rights reserved.

Abbreviations	
ANA	antinuclear antibodies
BLEC	benign lymphoepithelial cyst
CT	computed tomography
FNA	fine needle aspiration
HIV	human immunodeficiency virus
MALT	mucosa-associated lymphoid tissue
MRI	magnetic resonance imaging
NTM	nontuberculous mycobacteria
PCR	polymerase chain reaction
RA	rheumatoid arthritis
RAI	radioactive iodine
SLE	systemic lupus erythematosus
SMG	submandibular gland
SSS	jögren's Syndrome

SIALOLITHIASIS

Sialolithiasis is an obstructive disease of the salivary gland characterized by occlusion of the salivary ducts by calculus or stone. The incidence in the general population has been reported to be 1.2% and occurs predominantly in the submandibular gland (80%–90% of all sialoliths) as opposed to the parotid gland (5%–20% of all sialoliths).[1,2] These sialoliths may vary in size, from less than 1 mm to multiple centimeters; most are 3–7 mm in size. The most common location for salivary stones is in the hilum (proximal duct system), followed by the distal two-thirds of the ductal system. Rarely are these stones found within the salivary gland parenchyma.[1]

The etiology of these stones is not entirely clear and may be attributed to bacteria, foreign bodies, or "microliths" as the initial nidus over which sialoliths develop, while other theories note trauma as a possible cause.[3]

Clinical Presentation

Clinical presentation of sialolithiasis is varied. The typical patient with sialolithiasis presents with chronic, intermittent salivary gland swelling which resolves spontaneously. This swelling may be painful or painless, or may not be present at all. Usually, swelling occurs with meals. With complete obstruction of the ducts, patients may develop episodes of acute sialadenitis with an enlarged and exquisitely painful gland, purulent secretions, and even formation of an abscess (**Fig. 1** and Video 1). Predisposing conditions include Sjogren's syndrome, diabetes mellitus, dehydration, gout, autoimmune disease, medications lowering salivary gland production (such as anticholinergics), or tobacco.[2,3]

On physical examination, particular attention must be directed to openings of all four salivary ducts; not just the affected gland(s). Examination of the site of the papilla, its patency, and the quality of saliva are all important for surgical planning, based judgment and expertise. This will determine if the papilla will be easy to navigate with standard dilation techniques or if the surgeon should plan ahead of time for a floor of mouth exploration and sialodochoplasty for endoscopic access. Bimanual massage of the salivary gland is a necessary part of any salivary gland examination; sometimes, the sialolith may be palpated. During massage of the salivary glands, difficulty identifying the papilla or inability to express saliva may indicate a complete obstruction of the duct. Purulent fluid expressed from the ducts, erythema, induration, or tenderness to palpation would indicate an acute sialadenitis, for which active surgical intervention or endoscopic intervention is usually contraindicated. In-office sonography may be

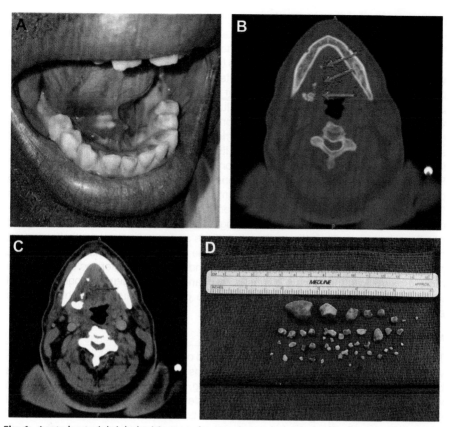

Fig. 1. Acute bacterial sialadenitis secondary to obstructive sialadenitis. (*A*) Enlarged and in-flamed right submandibular duct with purulence exuding from the papilla (*B*) Axial computed tomography scan showing multiple sialoliths along the right submandibular duct. The bone window shown here is helpful for elucidating the size and number of sialoliths (*yellow arrow*) (*C*) The same axial computed tomography scan shown in soft tissue window, which is helpful for identifying ductal dilation (*green arrow*) D) Over 40 sialoliths were removed from this patient. Note their varying size and architecture, and note that not all were visualized with preoperative CT

used for "sono-palpation" to assess the location and mobility of the sialolith. Firm, fibrotic glands may be indicative of chronic sialadenitis. Bilateral disease or pathologic findings on physical examination are more indicative of a systemic disease, such as one of the inflammatory diseases described later in this discussion. It is important to note that a complete head and neck examination must be performed in these patients to rule out malignancy or neoplasms. Flexible laryngoscopy should be performed to evaluate the upper aerodigestive tract for a possible primary head and neck malignancy when there is a high clinical suspicion or if patients have risk factors for malignancy, even in patients presenting with classical symptoms of sialadenitis.

Imaging

Various imaging modalities may be used to localize and characterize sialoliths in the office. Ultrasonography carries the advantage of being inexpensive, readily available, repeatable, noninvasive, and nonradiating.[3] As mentioned previously, it may be used in the clinic as an adjunct to the physical examination and in the operating room as well for the localization and confirmation of removal of all pathology. Its disadvantages are that false negatives may result in instances of small stones in nondilated salivary gland ducts; stones lesser than 2–3 mm in diameter can be missed on ultrasound.[2,4] Another potential disadvantage of ultrasound is that it is operator dependent. Ideally, surgeon-performed ultrasound has the greatest value in terms of efficiency of care, as it provides real-time information to the surgeon both in the clinic and in the operating room. Computerized tomography (CT) carries the advantages of being able to detect stones as small as 1 mm in size; however, its disadvantages are that it is a poor imaging modality for assessing for ductal dilation and carries a risk of radiation exposure.[4] Furthermore, CT is static, meaning that stones may relocate by the time that therapy is pursued. Another disadvantage with CT imaging is the presence of dental artifacts from prior dental procedures that can often mask pathology within the duct—especially in the distal duct. Conventional sialography is not as commonly performed but has the advantage of identifying ductal stenosis and may be therapeutic if sufficient dilation of the duct allows for the passage of the stone.[4] However, it also carries the risk of irradiation, possible ductal perforation, and the possibility of pushing the stone more proximally in the gland.[3] Magnetic resonance (MR) sialography can be helpful when there is a concern for another, separate pathology (such as a tumor) but is expensive and time-consuming.[4]

Management

Traditional management of sialolithiasis is based on the presence of symptoms. If salivary stones are asymptomatic, in many situations they can be observed until patients become symptomatic, causing repeated swelling, pain, or acute infections. In patients who are symptomatic, treatment options include conservative therapy with medical management consisting of appropriate broad-spectrum antibiotics, anti-inflammatory medications, and at times oral steroids. In addition, conservative measures are instituted that include hydration, gland massage, and sialagogues. Medical management is often used to quell an acute infection until definitive therapy with surgical intervention is planned. Historically, surgical intervention mainly included gland excision, which often required complete removal of the submandibular or parotid gland. In more favorable cases, whereby the stone or stenosis is located distally such that it could be accessed through the mouth, a transoral stone removal or repair of the stenosis is possible. However, gland removal is quite morbid. In addition to the complications associated with surgical procedures in general, specific complications with regards to salivary gland surgery include sialocele formation, recurrent symptoms or pathology from residual gland or duct, and injury to important nerves such as the hypoglossal nerve, lingual nerve, facial nerve, and marginal mandibular nerve. With parotid gland surgery specifically, Frey's syndrome, great auricular nerve paresis or palsy, and facial contour defects are possible.

Sialendoscopy is a relatively novel method of evaluating salivary duct pathology via direct visualization of the ducts (**Figs. 2** and **3**). This should be considered for any patient with sialolithiasis and for recurrent swelling of salivary glands without a specific etiology, especially swelling that is associated with meals and concerning obstructive pathology. One of the main advantages of sialendoscopy is its minimally invasive and low-risk nature with regards to major nerve damage, infection, hemorrhage, or dehiscence of an incision that is typically associated with external surgery. Endoscopy can be combined with transoral and external procedures to facilitate the management of stones and stenosis permitting gland preservation; these procedures are called

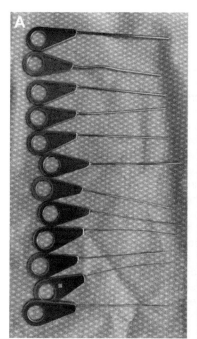
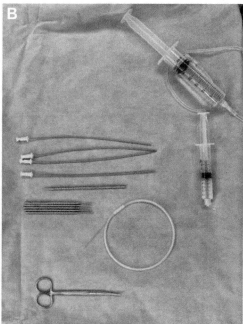

Fig. 2. Basic setup for salivary duct dilation. (*A*) Marchal salivary punctual dilators increase in size. Size 0000 is the smallest dilator and size 8 is the largest. (*B*) Mayo setup with useful instruments for sialendoscope (clockwise from the top); LUER-lock adapter and irrigation for sialendoscope, guidewire, scissors, metal salivary dilators, and hollow Cook dilators (Cook Medical, Bloomington, IL).

"hybrid" or "combined approach" procedures. Contraindications to sialendoscopy include acute sialadenitis and medical issues that would preclude general anesthesia. In cases of the former, medical therapy with antibiotics is preferred to treat the acute infection, as the risk of perforation of the salivary ducts is higher during episodes of acute infection and inflammation.[2] In cases of the latter, observation, and conservative management may be sufficient to subdue symptoms.

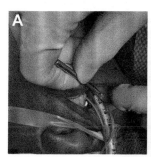
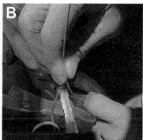
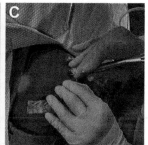

Fig. 3. Sialendoscope technique. (*A*) Salivary dilator used to dilate the right parotid papilla. (*B*) Cook dilator (Cook Medical, Bloomington, IL) used to further dilate papilla and duct prior to the introduction of sialendoscope. The advantage of this dilator is that it is hollow, so it may be inserted over a guidewire, (*C*) 1.1 mm sialendoscope inserted in left Stensen's duct and parotid gland. Note the transillumination over the left face.

ACUTE SUPPURATIVE (BACTERIAL) SIALADENITIS

Inflammation of the salivary glands is known as sialadenitis, and this can be further delineated into acute and chronic sialadenitis. Acute sialadenitis tends to be related to microbial pathogens, such as bacteria or viruses, while chronic sialadenitis tends to be associated with systemic diseases, many of which are described later in this article. In this section we will discuss acute bacterial sialadenitis; granulomatous conditions and viral etiologies will be discussed later in this article.

In instances of salivary gland obstruction, acute onset of inflammatory symptoms may occur. This may take the form of obstructive sialolithiasis, as described previously, but may also occur in the setting of other obstructive pathologies such as duct stenosis.[5] Clinical presentation is typical for unilateral enlargement of a single salivary gland with exquisite tenderness, overlying skin changes such as erythema and induration, and sometimes constitutional symptoms (eg, fevers, chills).[5] Risk factors for this condition include previously known ductal obstruction (eg, sialoliths), medications that decrease salivary excretion (eg, anticholinergics), dehydration, xerostomia, hypothyroidism, Sjogren's disease, and poor oral hygiene.[5] Physical examination is remarkable for marked enlargement of a salivary gland with trismus and extreme tenderness to the area.[2,5] Sometimes, purulent drainage can be expressed from the salivary duct during massage of the affected gland. Sometimes, fluctuance may be appreciated in the presence of an abscess, and stones may be palpated in the ducts if they are in the distal ductal system. The most common pathogen is *Staphylococcus aureus* (50%–90%), although other organisms including Streptococcus spp. and Haemophilus spp. have been identified and isolated as well.[5] Imaging is not always necessary but may be helpful in identifying etiology, sites of ductal obstruction, and localizing and mapping the extent of the abscesses, if present.[2] Treatment is medical in nature and consists of a combination of antibiotics covering gram-positive and anaerobic organisms, as well as conservative measures such as adequate hydration, salivary gland massage, warm compresses, sialagogues, and oral hygiene.[5]

Surgical intervention is usually not required except in instances of abscess formation or failure to respond to medical management.[5] Frequently, an inpatient admission with intravenous antibiotics will be necessary to help calm an acute episode. If the patient does not respond to therapy and there is a distal and easily accessible obstruction, a transoral approach and simple sialodochotomy to remove the stone and relieve the obstruction is a reasonable option. In the authors' experience (although normally contraindicated in this clinical scenario) an endoscopy of the inflamed duct under controlled settings with low-pressure irrigation can be considered with the intention to merely wash out the duct with antibiotic and/or steroid irrigation. This can significantly help in reducing pain, which in turn makes it possible for the patient to transition to oral medication, and thus possibly leading to earlier discharge. An endoscopic washout tends to expedite the clinical progress; however, physical examination findings such as gland swelling and induration may persist. These generally take weeks to resolve, with a more natural progression than one would expect. In episodes of recurrent acute sialadenitis, investigation into the etiology of the recurrent duct obstruction may be pursued after the acute infection has resolved.

VIRAL INFECTIONS OF SALIVARY GLANDS
Human Immunodeficiency Virus

The human immunodeficiency virus (HIV) is associated with multiple different disease processes involving the salivary glands. As such, the term "HIV-associated salivary gland disease" has historically been used to refer to this diffuse enlargement and inflammation of the salivary glands in the setting of HIV infection. The specific etiologies include conditions such as benign lymphoepithelial lesions, reactive lymphadenopathy, sialadenitis, mycobacterial infections, neoplasms (eg, Kaposi sarcoma), and a sicca-type inflammatory syndrome.[6] The parotid gland is the most common salivary gland involved, encompassing 1% to 10% of HIV-infected patients.[7] This parotid swelling is generally due to the development of multiple benign lesions within the glands. There are subtle differences in the specific histopathology of these various conditions, reflected by the myriad nomenclature used to describe them, including: benign lymphoepithelial cysts (BLECs), benign lymphoepithelial lesions (BLELs), AIDS-related lymphadenopathy, cystic lymphoid hyperplasia, and diffuse infiltrative lymphocytosis syndrome (DILS).[7,8] For purposes of this publication, these lesions will heretofore be referred to as BLECs. The high propensity for parotid involvement is thought to be related to the unique architecture of the parotid gland, with foci of lymphoid tissue interspersed within glandular tissue.[9] Some postulate that the incomplete ductal obstruction caused by this lymphoid hyperplasia within the gland causes epithelial cysts.[8] Disease of the salivary glands often occurs early in the HIV disease course, oftentimes preceding AIDS.[6] In fact, identification of these lymphoepithelial lesions is so uncommon in patients without HIV that their presence necessitates evaluation for HIV.[7,10]

Patients with HIV-SGD present with nontender glandular swelling that is bilateral in 80% of cases and involves multiple salivary glands in 90% of cases.[10] Patients also frequently report xerostomia, and cervical lymphadenopathy is commonly present. These lesions are readily identified on ultrasound, CT, and MRI, all of which demonstrate thin-walled cystic cavities with associated cervical lymphadenopathy.[10] Fine-needle aspiration (FNA) has a role in ruling out another salivary gland pathology, as will be described later in discussion.

A variety of treatment modalities for BLECs exist. On the conservative side of the spectrum, close observation is a reasonable option, as these lesions are benign by nature.[7,11] However, routine surveillance is crucial. While the association between BLECs and malignant transformation has not been identified, the HIV population, in general, is at higher risk for malignant diseases, such as EBV-associated malignant B-cell carcinoma.[10] As such, monitoring for any acute enlargement of the salivary glands is crucial, and any significant clinical or radiographic change warrants FNA to rule out other malignancy.

Medical therapy includes antivirals, which have demonstrated varied efficacy.[7]

Sclerotherapy with doxycycline has been shown to have some efficacy, if only in the short term.[9] Doxycycline has a low pH and is thought to induce an inflammatory response within the salivary glands, thus provoking secondary adhesions and obliteration of the cysts.[12] Notably, it does not seem to affect the difficulty of future parotidectomy should surgical intervention be required at a future date.[7] Some patients elect for repeated aspiration, which particularly is effective for the management of the cosmetic sequelae of HIV-SGD and carries the added benefit of allowing for concomitant FNA. However, cysts reaccumulate quickly within a matter of weeks, which may be burdensome as a long-term therapy.[7] Sodium morrhuate, a detergent sclerosant, has also been used for injection sclerotherapy with a 91.5% reduction in cyst size. This procedure is conducted in the operating room; side effects include postoperative edema and tenderness at the injection site. Fagan and colleagues have evaluated the use of alcohol injection sclerotherapy as a feasible, low-cost, outpatient option for treating HIV-related cystic disease.[12] More aggressive treatment includes radiation therapy and surgical excision of salivary glands. While low-dose radiation therapy shows efficacy in the reduction of parotid gland size, it is associated with undesirable side effects, including xerostomia and mucositis, and would make for future surgical excision of these glands technically more difficult.[7,10] Surgical excision is not a favorable option, as the bilateral and progressive nature of this disease would require multiple procedures with a significant risk of facial nerve injury and inability to completely treat the disease.[10] As such, surgery and radiation are reserved for late-stage HIV-SGD that has not responded to more conservative treatment modalities.[7]

Mumps

Mumps is a common childhood disease that is classically characterized by the bilateral swelling of the parotid glands. It represents the most common cause of parotid swelling in pediatric patients.[13] This nonsuppurative sialadenitis is caused by the paramyxovirus, which is a highly contagious RNA virus spread primarily via salivary secretions or respiratory droplets. The virus primarily affects the glandular epithelium, invading the ductal epithelium of the parotid gland and resulting in periductal interstitial edema and local inflammation.[14] After entering the upper respiratory tract, the incubation period is roughly 2 to 3 weeks.[15] Symptoms begin with a viral prodrome, consisting of fever, arthralgia, malaise, anorexia, and headache. Thereafter, patients then typically develop the classic painful parotid swelling over the subsequent 2 to 3 days. This swelling persists for roughly 1 to 2 weeks and is associated with otalgia, trismus, and odynophagia.[15] The parotid glands usually exhibit firm, nonpitting edema without warmth or overlying erythema. It is not uncommon for symptoms to begin with only one gland, followed by the enlargement of the contralateral gland days later. In more rare cases (<10% of infections), the submandibular or sublingual glands are also involved. Complications of mumps include meningoencephalitis, orchitis, pancreatitis, and nephritis.[13] After the initiation of the mumps vaccination program in the US in 1967, mumps cases decreased from 152,209 in 1968 to 231 in 2003. However, mumps cases and outbreaks continue to be reported, mostly in young adults and unvaccinated populations. Consequently, a history of vaccination is imperative when evaluating a patient who presents with diffuse bilateral parotid gland swellings.[16] Diagnosis of mumps is confirmed by laboratory testing, which predominantly consists of viral serology (IgM, IgG) but also includes the detection of mumps RNA via RT-PCR.[17] Patients typically exhibit normal white blood cell and differential counts, and in the setting of parotid involvement, serum amylase may be elevated.[14] Management includes mostly supportive care, as there is no specific antiviral therapy currently used against the paramyxovirus. This includes nonsteroidal anti-inflammatory drugs, antipyretics, bed rest, oral hygiene, and adequate hydration. As alluded to previously, vaccination is highly effective in the prevention of mumps. In the US, this live attenuated vaccine is given as part of the measles–mumps–rubella (MMR) vaccine series.[18]

GRANULOMATOUS INFECTIONS OF SALIVARY GLANDS
Tuberculous Mycobacterial Disease

Tuberculosis localized to the salivary glands is quite rare. Tuberculosis is uncommon in developed countries, and extrapulmonary tuberculosis only accounts for approximately 20% of cases, with cervical lymphadenitis serving as the most common presentation of extrapulmonary tuberculosis.[19–21] Furthermore, tuberculous salivary disease has myriad clinical presentations, thus complicating diagnosis. However, when primary tuberculosis infection of the salivary glands occurs, it generally affects the parotid glands and is more common in older children and adults.[20] Pathogenesis of this disease remains incompletely understood but is thought to spread via three main pathways: (1) direct spread from the oral cavity via glandular ductal system, or (2) hematogenous spread, or (3) ascending infection via lymphatics.[19–22] As mentioned previously, the clinical presentation of primary salivary gland tuberculosis is varied and can mimic other salivary gland diseases. One presentation consists of an indolent, chronic, slow-growing lesion mimicking a neoplasm. A second presentation mimics that of acute sialadenitis or abscess with diffuse inflammation and glandular edema. During both presentations, constitutional symptoms are often absent and cervical lymphadenopathy may not be present. Other presentations include fistula formation or, even more rarely, facial nerve paralysis.[19] Image modalities for the radiographic evaluation of these lesions include ultrasound, CT, and MRI. The radiographic findings are usually nonspecific, and again may take multiple forms, ranging from diffuse enlargement and homogenous enhancement with the involvement of lymph nodes to the development of discrete rim-enhancing lesions with central lucency.[20] Fine-needle aspiration cytology is perhaps the most useful approach for establishing diagnosis, with additional techniques such as Ziehl–Neelsen staining, culture, and PCR evaluation used to support the diagnosis.[19,20] Ideally, once the diagnosis is made, the preferred modality of treatment is medical, consisting of a combination of antitubercular agents.[19,21] Incisional biopsy or drainage is avoided, given the high risk for the development of cutaneous fistula.[19] If drainage is necessary, an incision in a nondependent site is ideal to lower the risk of creating a chronic draining wound or fistula. Abscesses associated with tuberculosis are typically not associated with the intense inflammation and pain usually seen with an infective process—hence the term, "cold abscess." In the presence of a cold abscess that does not conform to the expected clinical presentation of a conventional acute abscess, tuberculosis should be considered in the differential diagnosis.

Nontuberculous Mycobacterial Disease

Over the last several years, nontuberculous mycobacteria (NTM) have become an increasingly important pathogen implicated in cervicofacial lymphadenitis. As the term would indicate, NTM refers to the collective group of acid-fast bacilli that are not classified as Mycobacterium tuberculosis, which is important to distinguish due to the different treatment algorithms used for each. NTMs are omnipresent in the environment and may be isolated from a variety of soil, water, domestic wild animals, milk, and other food.[23] This group of pathogens typically affects small children, age 2 to 5, as well as immunocompromised patients. Recently, its incidence and severity have been rising, even in developed countries. Typical presentation is a pediatric patient with a unilateral rapidly progressing parotid or neck mass, frequently with violaceous discoloration. Patients often fail multiple courses of antibiotics before obtaining diagnosis, and fistulaization is not uncommon.[24] CT and MR imaging may be helpful for identifying and characterizing these granulomas and abscesses; these generally reveal low intensity, rim-enhancing masses. In contrast to conventional bacterial abscesses, there is often minimal or even absent fat stranding of surrounding soft tissue demonstrated on imaging.[23] Traditionally, surgical excision has been the predominant method of treatment, and has been described to have the highest cure rate.[24] However, in recent years, there has been an increasing amount of literature advocating for medical treatment alone or medical treatment in conjunction with surgery in hopes of achieving cure while avoiding the complications that may arise with surgical treatment.[23,25–27] Although this new ideology is gaining momentum, it is not yet well established, and surgical excision of the involved salivary glands and nodes remains the mainstay of management.[24,27]

OTHER GRANULOMATOUS DISEASES
Actinomycosis

Actinomycosis is a bacterial infection caused by *Actinomyces* spp., most classically *Actinomyces israelii*, which are gram-positive, nonacid fast, anaerobic commensurate bacteria within the oral cavity. They are commonly found in the tonsils and within dental tartar.[28] This chronic, suppurative, granulomatous infection is uncommon, but when it occurs, it preferentially affects the cervicofacial region, as it is usually odontogenic in origin.[28,29] This bacterium is found in normal flora and does not progress to infection in healthy tissue. It propagates and leads to pathologic infection in instances whereby tissue is compromised, either during trauma, decreased tissue oxygenation, or in diminished oxidation–reduction potential.[30] As such, risk factors for disease include oral trauma, maxillofacial trauma, surgery, radiation therapy, chronic head and neck infections (including tonsillitis), immunocompromised states (such as immunodeficiency, diabetes mellitus, or long term steroid use), or malnutrition.[28,30] However, it should be noted that most described infections occur in immunocompetent individuals.[28] Once inoculated, spread is typical via direct extension traversing multiple tissue planes. Hematogenous spread may occur but is more uncommon. In the setting of primary salivary gland actinomycosis, the likely method of inoculation is retrograde migration through the glandular ductal systems.[31]

Clinical presentation can be nonspecific and may take a slow, indolent course, making the diagnosis elusive. Cervicofacial actinomycosis typically starts as a soft tissue infection but can spread to adjacent structures, including bones and salivary glands.[28,30] Primary salivary gland actinomycosis is even more rare, but when it occurs, it typically involves the parotid gland.[27] This infection usually starts as a chronic suppurative or indurated mass around the ramus of the mandible.[28,30] On physical exam, nonspecific findings such as perimandibular or submandibular erythema, induration, or nodularity are appreciated. As time progresses, drainage or fistulous tracts may develop, sometimes with characteristic macroscopic sulfur granules appearing within the purulent drainage.[28,30] Cervical lymphadenopathy is rare, and if it develops, it may not do so until later in the disease course.[28,29]

Initial laboratory workup shows nonspecific signs of inflammation and infection, such as mild leukocytosis and elevated inflammatory markers (eg, C reactive protein, erythrocyte sedimentation rate).[30] Serology is not useful for identifying *Actinomyces* spp., although it may be helpful for ruling out other organisms. Ultrasound, CT, and MRI are often used in the workup of this disease but typically reveal nonspecific or even misleading findings. Imaging modalities may reveal a spectrum of findings and can be suggestive of nonspecific malignant, inflammatory, or even erosive processes.[28,30] Tissue culture is the most accurate and preferable form of diagnosis and is most easily facilitated via fine-needle aspiration (FNA) culture, although the specimen may take multiple weeks to grow and speciate.[28–30] Long-term penicillin remains the mainstay of antibiotic treatment.[27–30] Third-generation cephalosporins are useful in penicillin-allergic patients.[28] Surgery plays a role in many patients, usually in the setting of removal of fibrotic debris and sinus tracts, draining abscesses when present, and offering greater diagnostic yield when FNA is insufficient.[29]

Cat-Scratch Disease

Cat-scratch disease, caused by the intracellular fastidious gram-negative bacteria *Bartonella henselae*, is a common cause of cervicofacial lymphadenitis. The natural vector of these bacteria is the feline. This disease may occur in patients of all ages and may occur in either immunocompetent or immunocompromised patients.[32]

Patients typically present with a nontender, discolored papule approximately 3 to 10 days after contact with a cat.[33] Although a cat scratch or cat bite is not necessary for the transmission of this disease, it is often noted in the patient's history.[33,34] Patients then develop regional lymphadenopathy in the following 2 weeks that persists for weeks. 80% of patients will experience lymphadenopathy, which is the most common symptom.[33] The neck is the most common site of involvement; involvement of the parotid gland and the deep parotid space is rare.[34] In many instances, suppurative changes develop within these lymph nodes.[35] Imaging typically reveals nonspecific findings but may be helpful for localizing the affected lymph nodes, identifying abscesses, and monitoring disease. While PCR testing of a biopsied specimen is the most sensitive method of diagnosis, this technology is not always readily available. The mainstay of diagnosis remains serologic testing for antibodies against B henselae.[32,33] A variety of antibiotics such as macrolides (azithromycin), trimethoprim-sulfamethoxazole, and rifampin have been used to effectively treat this disease.[34] Beta-lactams and cephalosporins are ineffective.[35] Fine-needle aspiration or surgical debridement is seldom required, with roughly 10% of patients requiring surgical drainage of an abscess.[32,35]

NONINFECTIOUS INFLAMMATORY DISEASES OF SALIVARY GLANDS
Sjögren's Syndrome

Sjögren's syndrome (SS) is a chronic autoimmune disease of the exocrine glands of affected individuals. It can be primary or secondary: primary occurring when disease is present without other systemic autoimmune diseases, and secondary occurring in the presence of other autoimmune dysfunction, such as rheumatoid arthritis (RA) or systemic lupus erythematosus (SLE, or lupus). It is present in 6 out of 100,000 people, more common in the elderly, and 10 times as prevalent in women compared to men. Pathogenesis is not well understood, but B cells are thought to lay a key role in exocrine gland swelling and production of anti-SSA and anti-SSB autoantibodies.[36]

Reported symptoms on initial presentation are varied. Some patients exhibit mild symptoms that are not bothersome, while others with severe symptoms will have significant quality of life disturbances. The group of symptoms that can be categorized as sicca symptoms includes dry mouth, dysphagia, and dental caries resulting from xerostomia. Extreme symptoms may give patients the sensation of having "cotton mouth." Glandular swelling is often seen, with ranging severity from spontaneous resolution to painful, persistent swelling with nodular and indurated glands identified on examination. Late-stage SS may present with firm glands, purulent "tooth-paste" like secretions from the ducts, and irreversible changes in the glandular parenchyma such as multi-cystic disease and inflammatory intra- or periglandular lymphadenopathy.

There exist diagnostic criteria set forth by the Revised American European Consensus Group classification criteria for SS. Briefly, these include (1) ocular symptoms such as dry eyes requiring artificial tears, (2) oral symptoms such as salivary gland enlargement or xerostomia, (3) ocular signs including an abnormal Schirmer test, (4) salivary gland biopsy showing lymphocytic sialadenitis, (5) oral signs including abnormal salivary scintigraphy, and (6) identification of SSA and SSB autoantibodies.[37] The classical triad of symptoms in the sicca complex includes dry eyes, dry mouth, and salivary gland enlargement. In spite of several diagnostic tests and criteria, the formal diagnosis of SS is quite challenging. Many patients exhibit classical sicca symptoms yet may test negative for antibodies and may demonstrate unremarkable histopathology on minor salivary gland lip biopsies.

Salivary gland ultrasound is useful to assist in diagnosis.[38,39] The bilateral parotid and submandibular glands undergo an ultrasound in conjunction with the thyroid for comparison. A grading system exists to help with evaluation developed by Horcevar and colleagues (Table 1).[39] A total score greater than 14 has been associated with abnormal imaging, and greater than or equal to 17 associated with Sjögren's syndrome.[38–40]

Minor salivary gland biopsy can assist with diagnosis, especially in patients with negative anti-SSA and anti-SSB antibodies. The sensitivity and specificity are greater than 80% in most studies.[41] Minor salivary gland biopsies can be performed both at the time of an intervention for the salivary glands in the operating room, or even as an in-office procedure. The key to accurate diagnosis and successful surgery is achieving sufficient hemostasis and meticulously searching to isolate 5 to 6 minor salivary glands for evaluation. The authors find that an incision on the inner mucosal surface of the lower lip is cosmetically acceptable and provides great access for tissue diagnosis. A small 1.0–1.5 cm mucosal incision is required; sharp dissection is generally adequate for the remainder of the exposure and excision. Of note, the mucosa should be closed with an inverted 4-0 or 5-0 absorbable suture so that it is not bothersome to the patient.

There are several options for the treatment of Sjögren's syndrome. As one can imagine, medical management with a "salivary gland regimen" and medical therapy works well for early-stage SS. This "salivary gland regimen" includes aggressive hydration, smoking cessation, and salivary gland massage. For medical management, pilocarpine and other secretagogues are beneficial for symptomatic management. Steroids may help with glandular enlargement and systemic symptoms but have not been shown to significantly improve sicca symptoms. Immunosuppressive agents such as methotrexate and azathioprine can be used as well. Rituximab, a monoclonal antibody against the CD20 protein of B cells, has also shown efficacy.[37]

On the other hand, patients who present with chronic symptoms and near end-stage SS are challenging to manage. Early-stage SS responds well to medical management; sialendoscopy is a reasonable option as well to help endoscopically evaluate the ducts for stenosis, debris, and occasionally stones (Fig. 4). Endoscopic washouts with or without steroid infusion can help patients who present with glandular swelling or painful glands, as they can reduce gland size, improve facial contour, ameliorate pain, and reduce the frequency and intensity of acute flare-ups. However, this procedure does

Table 1 Salivary gland ultrasound	
Ultrasound Finding	**Scoring**
(1) Parenchymal echogenicity compared with thyroid parenchyma	0–1
(2) Homogeneity	0–3
(3) Presence of hypoechoic areas in parenchyma	0–3
(4) Presence of hyperechoic foci	0–3
• Parotid glands	0–1
• Submandibular glands	
(5) Clearness of the salivary gland border	0–3
Total	

This table demonstrates the scaling system developed by Hocevar et al. for salivary gland ultrasound. Each score of the five domains is added together. A score greater than 14 is associated with abnormal imaging and a score greater than or equal to 17 is associated with Sjögren's syndrome.

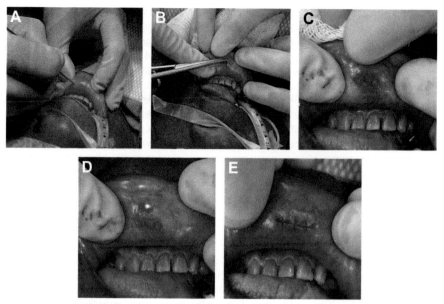

Fig. 4. Minor salivary gland biopsy. This figure depicts the operative steps for minor salivary gland biopsy. (*A*) 1 cm incision is made in the lower lip mucosa under tension. (*B*) A hemostat used to dissect the submucosal tissue to visualize the minor salivary glands (*C*) Minor salivary glands are exposed. These will protrude when placed under tension. (*D*) Minor salivary gland is removed and is placed next to the incision site, for comparison. These are sent for pathologic analysis. (*E*) The lower lip mucosal incision is closed with 4 to 0 Vicryl (Ethicon Inc., Cincinnati, OH) suture in an interrupted fashion, taking care to bury the knot.

not provide any long-term relief for sicca symptoms. It is also important to recognize that in end-stage SS, one must always have a high index of suspicion for the development of lymphoma, especially mucosa-associated lymphoid tissue (MALT) lymphoma).[42] Most patients with late-stage SS will undergo chronic surveillance with their rheumatologist, require frequent image-guided or open biopsies of their glands to rule out malignant change, and may occasionally benefit from an endoscopic intervention. Most likely, however, patients will need surgical extirpation of the affected glands.

Sarcoidosis

Sarcoidosis is a chronic granulomatous multi-system disorder, commonly affecting the lungs, but also can be noted to affect the salivary glands, particularly the parotid gland.[43–45] The disease pathogenesis is not completely understood but thought to start in the lungs and spread lymphatically to other sites.[43,44] Involvement of the salivary glands is relatively uncommon, affecting only about 6% of patients.[44] Most commonly seen in African American and female patients, it presents with painless swelling of the parotid glands, xerostomia, and less commonly facial nerve palsy.[43,44] A subset of patients present with uveoparotid fever (Heerfordt's syndrome) that consists of a complex collection of symptoms involving fever, parotid enlargement, uveitis, and facial nerve palsy. This facial nerve palsy is typically transient and due to the granulomatous infiltration of the nerve.[44] Generally, cranial neuropathy is indicative of a malignant process within the salivary glands and is a pathognomonic sign of advanced disease. Consequently, even though transient facial neuropathy may be a presentation of uveoparotid fever, it is imperative that malignancy remains on the differential diagnosis. If there is any clinical concern for malignancy, one should consider imaging and, if necessary, a guided diagnostic biopsy of the affected gland to both rule out a neoplastic process and confirm sarcoidosis histopathologically.

The gold standard for diagnosis of sarcoidosis is transbronchial lung biopsy or mediastinoscopy, achieving the diagnosis in 60% and 100% of patients, respectively. However, minor salivary gland biopsy is also a possible means of establishing the diagnosis, with a sensitivity of 18% to 41%.[46] The ease of minor salivary gland biopsy makes it an attractive alternative in the outpatient setting.[47] Histopathology of the involved salivary tissue shows noncaseating granulomas in the absence of obvious infection.[43–45] Laboratory values may demonstrate increased serum angiotensin-converting enzyme (ACE) and erythrocyte sedimentation rate (ESR) during active disease states.[43,45] Patients are typically treated with corticosteroids. Steroid-sparing treatment includes methotrexate and other immunosuppressive agents.[44,45]

IgG4-Related Disease

IgG4-related disease is a chronic disease that is immune mediated and affects multiple organ systems.[48–50] It has been shown to affect lacrimal and salivary glands as part of the disease spectrum. It has previously been described as Mikulicz's syndrome or Küttner tumor but is now recognized under the more broad term "IgG4-related disease."[49,50] Patients generally present with xerostomia and chronic sialadenitis. Unilateral or bilateral painless salivary gland enlargement is often encountered, most commonly involving the submandibular glands. Those individuals with major salivary gland disease are more likely to have multiorgan disease and higher disease activity. On CT imaging, major salivary glands may be enlarged and show diffuse homogenous enhancement. On laboratory analysis, patients demonstrate increased levels of IgG4 and IgE, and a quarter of patients are positive for rheumatoid factor and antinuclear antibodies (ANA).[48–50] Patients are typically anti-Ro/SSA and anti-La/SSB negative.[49,50] Incisional biopsy of the submandibular gland is useful and is routinely considered to establish a diagnosis. There have been case reports describing the use of minor salivary gland lip biopsy as a less invasive alternative to secure a diagnosis as an adjunct to clinical and laboratory work up.[51] Histopathologic analysis reveals IgG4 plasma cell infiltrates with fibrosis, obliterative phlebitis, and eosinophilia. Treatment consists of glucocorticoids and steroid-sparing agents such as azathioprine.[49,50] Like in Sjögren's syndrome, some patients may benefit from endoscopic intervention in addition to medical management to aid with pain and glandular swelling. However, the clinical features of a firm fibrotic gland, as can sometimes be expected with autoimmune sialadenitis, will unlikely change with endoscopic washout as can be sometimes expected with autoimmune sialadenitis.

Radioactive Iodine-Induced Sialadenitis

Radioactive iodine (RAI) is used for thyroid ablation in patients who suffer from Graves' disease, patients with toxic thyroid nodules, and more commonly patients with residual thyroid tissue after total thyroidectomy for differentiated thyroid cancer. However, RAI can have a detrimental impact on the salivary glands.[52–56] The mechanism of salivary gland damage is based on the activity of the sodium/potassium/chloride co-transporter, which enables the ductal cells to concentrate I-131 to approximately 30 to 40 times that of plasma concentrations. Because the ductal system may be affected by RAI in addition to salivary acini—as compared to external beam radiation, which tends to injury salivary acini—ductal strictures and obstructive sialadenitis can occur.

Parotid glands are more prone to RAI-induced injury as serous cells, which are predominant in the parotid, are more prone to injury from RAI concentration than mucus acini (found predominantly in the SMG).[52–55]

The incidence of RAI-induced sialadenitis is dose-dependent and ranges from 10% to 60%. A higher proportion of women are affected compared with men, perhaps due to the increased likelihood of thyroid pathology in women. Patients with RAI sialadenitis exhibit symptoms of obstructive sialadenitis and also chronic inflammatory disease characterized by glandular swelling, pain, and xerostomia. These symptoms may seem a few days to even months following RAI treatment.[52–54] Salivary gland swelling is a common symptom, but one that is not often discussed.[56] Consequently, many patients who have these symptoms do not report them. Counseling patients to report these symptoms and seek care for their salivary symptoms could result in earlier intervention with sialendoscopy and washout, and possibly delay late sequelae of RAI sialadenitis. However, there is not yet objective data to support this argument. On clinical examination, saliva may often be perceived as "ropy" and thick but not purulent. Diagnosis is mostly clinical but objective salivary flow rates can be measured and are reduced compared with controls.

Treatment is generally conservative, mimicking that of autoimmune sialadenitis with salivary gland hygiene, gland massages, hydration, and sialagogues.[54–56] With the advent of sialendoscopy, one can evaluate and manage obstructive strictures as well as offer washouts of the affected glands with either saline, steroids, antibiotics, or a combination thereof. Endoscopic findings commonly include debris, focal strictures, and evidence of chronic sialadenitis as seen by the loss of vascular markings in the ductal lumen.[54,55] Success rates with sialendoscopy vary from 50% to 100%.[55,56] In the author's own experience, 75% of patients have symptomatic relief. Success is gauged by the absence of symptoms or reduction in the intensity and frequency of recurring symptoms.

SALIVARY DUCT STENOSIS

Salivary duct stenosis is a relatively common disorder of the salivary glands and the second most common cause of obstructive sialadenitis after salivary stones. Stenosis is a consequence of several etiologies such as trauma to the duct, autoimmunity, calculi, or recurrent infections.[57] The diagnosis, classification, and management of stenoses have relevance for both obstructive and inflammatory ductal disease.

Patients typically present with glandular swelling and pain after meals or salivary stimulation.[57,58] No obstructive stones are seen on subsequent imaging, and 75% of patients with stenosis have parotid involvement.[58]

Ultrasound of the salivary glands, especially the parotid gland, can be helpful in the evaluation of ductal anomalies such as megaduct, webs, and kinking that can lead to duct stenosis.[59] Vitamin C can be used to elucidate the site of duct stenosis by dilating nonstenotic segments, especially in megaduct.[60,61] Stenosis can be evaluated radiographically with MR sialography, showing various types of stenosis which are characterized as either focal, multifocal, long segmental, or diffuse.[57]

Treatment options vary depending on patient presentation. For patients with asymptomatic or rarely symptomatic stenosis, conservative treatment with gland massage, anti-inflammatory medications, and occasional antibiotic treatment is recommended.[60]

Sialography-guided balloon dilation is a reasonable intervention early in the disease course, which is relatively efficient in relieving both patient symptoms and improving stenosis on subsequent imaging. However, as mentioned previously, this entity gives only an indirect view of the ductal system and is associated with radiation exposure; as such, it has largely fallen out of favor.[60]

Sialendoscopy is both a diagnostic tool and a first-line treatment option for obstructive salivary disease. There have been various grading systems described for stenosis. Lim and colleagues denote a grading system with Grade 1 representing inflammatory stenosis, grade 2 with fibrous narrowing less than 50%, and grade 3 with fibrous narrowing greater than 50%.[57] Hackman, and colleagues characterize stenosis similarly to the way tracheal stenosis is commonly graded: Grade 1 at 0% to 50% stenosis, grade 2 at 50% to 70% stenosis, grade 3 at 71% to 99% stenosis, and grade 4 with complete occlusive stenosis.[58] The location and length of the stenosis should be noted at well, as it is important to understand whether the stenosis occurs at the ostium, distal or proximal main duct, hilum, or within the gland.[58] During sialendoscopy, the ductal papilla can be gently dilated. The sialendoscope is advanced to visualize the stenotic areas (**Fig. 5**). These areas can then be gently dilated with dilators or saline infusion. Intraductal steroids can also be administered to assist with decreasing inflammation, as this has shown to improve outcomes.[57,60]

For Wharton's duct stenosis specifically, sialendoscopy with steroid irrigation, obturator dilation, and/or stent placement has efficacy in up to 50% to 80% of patients with a very high gland preservation rate. For ostial or distal stenosis, sialendoscopic techniques may be trailed at first to attempt gland preservation, but if this fails, transoral duct surgery or marsupialization of the duct has shown efficacy in resolving disease.[60,61] Different treatment algorithms exist depending on the location of the stenosis. For stenoses at the proximal duct or hilum, sialendoscopy with intervention or steroid irrigation should be the first procedure used after conservative therapy; however, if this fails one may consider transoral ductal surgery. If this still does not provide relief, Botox or submandibular gland excision should be considered. In cases of intraparenchymal stenosis, if the stenosis is visible, interventional sialendoscopy can be trialed. If this is unsuccessful, steroid irrigation is recommended. If this fails, gland excision or Botox should be considered. Traditionally, ductal ligation had been used, but this is no longer recommended, as this has shown to be successful in only 50% of patients.[60,61]

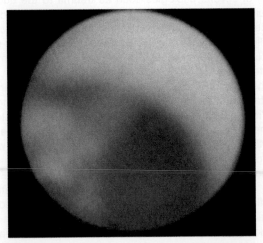

Fig. 5. Inflammatory salivary gland disease. Sialendoscopic view of salivary duct noting white debris within the ductal lumen, which can be seen in inflammatory salivary disease.

This treatment algorithm is similar for Stensen's duct stenosis, once again based on the location of stenosis which is characterized as either (1) papilla/distal duct, (2) middle and proximal duct/hilum, and (3) intraparenchymal stenosis. For patients with intraparenchymal stenosis, a combined approach can be considered with the resection of the stenotic segment and an interposition vein graft.[60,61]

Selection of treatment modality also depends on the disease severity. It has been shown that patients with less severe stenosis on MR sialography or sialendoscopy has better clinical outcomes with symptom control after sialendoscopy.[57] There is a paucity of literature on the management of severe stenosis in more distal areas of the parotid duct, such as whereby the duct traverses the masseter muscle (Reed). Reed and colleagues describe an open parotidectomy approach through modified Blair incision to isolate the stenotic portion of the duct, resecting the stenotic segment, and placing an interposition vein graft between the proximal and distal Stensen duct segments.[58]

Special consideration for intervention is given to patients with Stensen's megaduct. This is classified as a parotid duct larger than 10 mm proximal to the stenotic segment. This can cause obstructive symptoms as well as cosmetic concerns due to external visibility of the ductal dilation (**Fig. 6** and Video 3).[62] Transoral pull through sialodochoplasty can be performed to relieve the obstruction. In this instance, an obturator is placed in the duct and the mucosa surrounding the duct is incised. The megaduct is delivered into the oral cavity. The scarred portion of the duct is excised, and the megaduct mucosa is sutured to the buccal mucosa to create a new ostium. This can improve both patient symptoms and quality of life.[62]

SIALADENOSIS

Sialadenosis is a chronic non–immune-related disorder of the salivary glands.[63] It is characterized by diffuse glandular swelling, usually of the parotids, with occasional facial pain and possibly sialorrhea. The pathogenesis is not completely understood but thought to be related to the autonomic dysfunction of the myoepithelial cells and enlargement of the acini due to decreased exocytosis.[63,64] It may be seen with other chronic illnesses such as diabetes, alcohol consumption, malnutrition, or eating disorders.[63,65] On examination, patients have glandular enlargement.[63] For diagnosis, there must not be signs of inflammatory disease, stones, or strictures, as this is often a diagnosis of exclusion.

Imaging can sometimes be useful in these patients, depending on the etiology. Sialography is helpful to rule out obstruction. CT imaging typically shows glandular

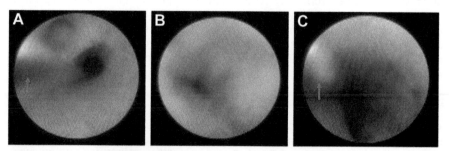

Fig. 6. Salivary duct stenosis. (A) Normal appearance of salivary duct with guidewire (*yellow arrow*) also in place during sialendoscopy. (B) Salivary ductal stricture. (C) Salivary duct stricture with guidewire (*yellow arrow*) passed through stricture.

enlargement with normal-appearing parotid intensity, and later in the disease, fatty infiltration. Fine-needle aspiration of salivary glands in this population can help to rule in the disease. This shows enlarged acini and acinar cells, usually 2 to 3 times the normal size, with basally displaced nuclei.[66]

Treatment is aimed at reversing the underlying chronic illness which predisposes patients to the disease, in addition to conservative treatment with heat application and glandular massage. Traditional surgical options included glandular excision.[66] However, more recent interventions aimed at preserving the salivary glands include Botox injections and tympanic neurectomy, both aimed at reducing parasympathetic input to the affected glands.[63]

FREY SYNDROME (AURICULOTEMPORAL SYNDROME)

Frey syndrome, also known as gustatory sweating, is a condition characterized by facial sweating and skin flushing over the parotid region induced by mastication or salivary stimulation. This can occur after trauma or salivary gland surgery, especially parotid surgery.[67,68] This is mediated by parasympathetic nerves from the auriculo-temporal nerve, which is a branch of the mandibular branch of the trigeminal nerve (V3).

When these normal innervations are disrupted during trauma or surgery, there is aberrant regeneration and reinnervation of these nerves with the sympathetic nerves controlling the exocrine sweat glands and venous plexus of the skin.[68] If symptoms occur, they typically are manifested 11 months following surgery. Incidence after paro-tidectomy ranges from 12.5% to 98%, but only around 12% to 30% are symptom-atic.[68,69] A positive starchiodine test may be useful in making diagnosis, although this has been shown to be positive in up to 98% of patients—even those who are asymptomatic. Frey syndrome has been cited as a major cause of patient morbidity and dissatisfaction.[68]

Various therapies are available to treat this disorder. This includes botulinum toxin A injection into the dermis of the affected areas, which essentially serves as an anti-cholinergic agent to block neurotransmission of the misaligned neural pathway.[69] The primary surgical intervention pursued in these cases is the placement of interpo-sition graft between the parotid bed and overlying skin. Options for graft material in these situations include acellular dermal matrix placement, temporoparietal fascia interposition, superficial musculoaponeurotic system flap, free fat graft, or sterno-cleidomastoid (SCM) muscle transfer.[67–69] To perform the SCM interposition graft, the mastoid portion of the SCM must first be divided. The anterior portion of the mus-cle is dissected free from the inferior aspect in a caudal-to-cranial direction, leaving the muscle attached superiorly. Dissection is limited to the anterior/superficial aspect of the SCM to avoid injury to the spinal accessory nerve. The inferior portion of the SCM that is dissected free is then transposed into the parotid bed wound and sutured in place.[70,71] There are limited randomized control studies comparing these methods to one another on Frey syndrome prevention, but all are viable options to reduce the incidence.[68–71]

SUMMARY

A large number of the above nonneoplastic salivary gland conditions have been known and studied for years without many advances in the management of these conditions. Clinical presentation can be quite similar across different diseases, despite their myriad etiologies, and treatment often begins with conservative therapies such as gland massage, hydration, and secretagogues. Historically, advanced disease necessitated gland extirpation without efficacious options for gland-preserving treatment. However, over the last 20 years, there has been significant progress in both medical and surgical modalities that effectively ameliorate patients' symptoms without sacrificing the salivary glands, thus avoiding the multifarious risks associated with surgical excision. As both new technology and improved technical skills of the physician who employs it continues to progress, the field will continue to see improved treatment outcomes, patient satisfaction, and cost-effective care.

CLINICS CARE POINTS

- During the examination of patients in the office with sialolithiasis, ultrasound may be a helpful adjunctive tool to both identify the specific location of the sialolith within the duct and to assess its mobility, which may assist in surgical decision making.

- In patients admitted to the hospital with acute sialadenitis who do not respond initially to therapy, minimal endoscopic intervention and ductal irrigation with antibiotics and steroids may improve short-term symptoms, allowing for earlier discharge and improved tolerance of oral antibiotics.

- Identification of lymphoepithelial lesions within the salivary glands necessitates evaluation and workup for HIV.

- If drainage of a salivary gland abscess in a patient with suspected tuberculosis is necessary, an incision in a nondependent site is ideal to lower the risk of creating a chronic draining wound or fistula.

- When working up patients with suspected Sjögren's disease who have negative anti-SSA and anti-SSB, consider a minor salivary gland biopsy to aid in yielding a histopathologic diagnosis.

DISCLOSURE

The authors have nothing to disclose.

SUPPLEMENTARY DATA

Supplementary data related to this article can be found online at https://doi.org/10.1016/j.suc.2022.01.001.

REFERENCES

1. Sigismund PE, Zenk J, Koch M, et al. Nearly 3,000 salivary stones: some clinical and epidemiologic aspects. Laryngoscope 2015;125(8):1879–82.
2. Hernandez S, Busso C, Walvekar RR. Parotitis and Sialendoscopy of the Parotid Gland. Otolaryngologic Clin North Am 2016;49(2):381–93.
3. Marchal F, Dulguerov P. Sialolithiasis Management: The State of the Art. Arch Otolaryngology–Head Neck Surg 2003;129(9):951–6.
4. Afzelius P, Nielsen MY, Ewertsen C, et al. Imaging of the major salivary glands. Clin Physiol Funct Imaging 2016;36(1):1–10.
5. Wilson KF, Meier JD, Ward PD. Salivary Gland Disorders. AFP 2014;89(11):882–8.
6. Schiødt M, Dodd CL, Greenspan D, et al. Natural history of HIV-associated salivary gland disease. Oral Surg Oral Med Oral Pathol 1992;74(3):326–31.
7. Dave SP, Pernas FG, Roy S. The Benign Lymphoepithelial Cyst and a Classification System for Lymphocytic Parotid Gland Enlargement in the Pediatric HIV Population. The Laryngoscope 2007;117(1):106–13.

8. Mandel L, Hong J. HIV-associated parotid lymphoepithelial cysts. The J Am Dental Assoc 1999;130(4):528–32.

9. Marsot-Dupuch K, Quillard J, Meyohas MC. Head and neck lesions in the immunocompromised host. Eur Radiol 2004;14(Suppl 3):E155–67.

10. Shanti RM, Aziz SR. HIV-associated Salivary Gland Disease. Oral Maxillofacial Surg Clin North America 2009;21(3):339–43.

11. Mandel L. Salivary gland disorders. Med Clin North Am 2014;98(6):1407–49.

12. Meyer E, Lubbe DE, Fagan JJ. Alcohol sclerotherapy of human immunodeficiency virus related parotid lymphoepithelial cysts. The J Laryngol Otology. 2009;123:422–5.

13. Brook I. Diagnosis and Management of Parotitis. Arch Otolaryngology–Head Neck Surg 1992;118(5):469–71.

14. Hviid A, Rubin S, Mühlemann K. Mumps. Lancet. 2008;371(9616):932–44.

15. Su SB, Chang HL, Chen KT. Current Status of Mumps Virus Infection: Epidemiology, Pathogenesis, and Vaccine. Int J Environ Res Public Health 2020;17(5):1686.

16. Mumps CDC. Cases and Outbreaks. Centers for Disease Control and Prevention. 2021. Available at: https://www.cdc.gov/mumps/outbreaks.html. Accessed December 14, 2021.

17. Maillet M, Bouvat E, Robert N, et al. Mumps outbreak and laboratory diagnosis. J Clin Virol 2015;62:14–9.

18. Clarkson E, Mashkoor F, Abdulateef S. Oral Viral Infections. Dent Clin North Am 2017;61:351–63.

19. Medeiros N, Oliveira P, Larangeiro J, et al. Tuberculosis as a differential diagnosis of salivary gland malignancy. BMJ Case Rep CP 2020;13(8):e233616.

20. Vyas S, Kaur N, Yadav TD, et al. Tuberculosis of parotid gland masquerading parotid neoplasm. Natl J Maxillofac Surg 2012;3(2):199–201.

21. Cataño JC, Robledo J. Tuberculous Lymphadenitis and Parotitis. Microbiol Spectr 2016;4(6). 4.6.22.

22. Maurya MK, Kumar S, Singh HP, et al. Tuberculous parotitis: A series of eight cases and review of literature. Natl J Maxillofac Surg 2019;10(1):118–22.

23. Bonali M, Mattioli F, Alicandri-Ciufelli M, et al. Atypical mycobacteriosis involving parotid and para-retropharyngeal spaces. Eur Arch Otorhinolaryngol 2016;273(11):4031–3.

24. Koo EY, Maksimoski MT, Herron MM, et al. Surgical management of parotid non-tuberculous mycobacteria lymphadenitis in children: A pediatric tertiary-care hospital's experience. Int J Pediatr Otorhinolaryngol 2021;151:110960.

25. Kay-Rivest E, Bouhabel S, Oughton MT, et al. Medical Management for the Treatment of Nontuberculous Mycobacteria Infection of the Parotid Gland: Avoiding Surgery May Be Possible. Case Rep Med 2016;2016:4324525.

26. Zimmermann P, Tebruegge M, Curtis N, et al. The management of non-tuberculous cervicofacial lymphadenitis in children: A systematic review and meta-analysis. J Infect 2015;71(1):9–18.

27. Varghese BT, Sebastian P, Ramachandran K, et al. Actinomycosis of the parotid masquerading as malignant neoplasm. BMC Cancer 2004;4:7.

28. Lancella A, Abbate G, Foscolo A, et al. Two unusual presentations of cervicofacial actinomycosis and review of the literature. Acta Otorhinolaryngol Ital 2008;28(2):89–93.

29. Volante M, Contucci A, Fantoni M, et al. Cervicofacial actinomycosis: still a difficult differential diagnosis. Acta Otorhinolaryngol Ital 2005;25(2):116–9.

30. Karanfilian KM, Valentin MN, Kapila R, et al. Cervicofacial actinomycosis. Int J Dermatol 2020;59(10):1185–90.
31. Bartels LJ, Vrabec DP. Cervicofacial actinomycosis: a variable disorder. Arch Otolaryngol 1978;705.
32. Ridder GJ, Boedeker CC, Technau-Ihling K, et al. Role of Cat-Scratch Disease in Lymphadenopathy in the Head and Neck. Clin Infect Dis 2002;35(6):643–9.
33. Ridder GJ, Boedeker CC, Technau-Ihling K, et al. Cat-scratch disease: Otolaryngologic manifestations and management. Otolaryngol Head Neck Surg 2005; 132(3):353–8.
34. Hollitt A, Buttery J, Carr J, et al. Cat scratch disease of the parotid gland. Arch Dis Child 2016;101(1):63–4.
35. Munson PD, Boyce TG, Salomao DR, et al. Cat-scratch disease of the head and neck in a pediatric population: Surgical indications and outcomes. Otolaryngol Head Neck Surg 2008;139(3):358–63.
36. Tian Y, Yang H, Liu N, et al. Advances in Pathogenesis of Sjögren's Syndrome. J Immunol Res 2021;2021:e5928232.
37. Fox RI, Fox CM, Gottenberg JE, et al. Treatment of Sjögren's syndrome: current therapy and future directions. Rheumatology (Oxford) 2021;60(5):2066–74.
38. Lee KA, Lee SH, Kim HR. Ultrasonographic Changes of Major Salivary Glands in Primary Sjögren's Syndrome. J Clin Med 2020;9(3):E803.
39. Hocevar A, Rainer S, Rozman B, et al. Ultrasonographic changes of major salivary glands in primary Sjögren's syndrome. Evaluation of a novel scoring system. Eur J Radiol 2007;63(3):379–83.
40. Rasmussen A, Ice JA, Li H, et al. Comparison of the American-European Consensus Group Sjogren's syndrome classification criteria to newly proposed American College of Rheumatology criteria in a large, carefully characterised sicca cohort. Ann Rheum Dis 2014;73(1):31–8.
41. Edelstein R, Kilipiris GE, Machalekova K, et al. Accuracy of minor salivary gland biopsy in the diagnosis of Sjögren syndrome. Bratisl Lek Listy 2021;122(7): 454–60.
42. Vasaitis L, Nordmark G, Theander E, et al. Population-based study of patients with primary Sjögren's syndrome and lymphoma: lymphoma subtypes, clinical characteristics, and gender differences. Scand J Rheumatol 2020;49(3):225–32.
43. Rao V, Curran J, Blair EA, et al. Salivary glands sarcoidosis. Oper Tech Otolaryngology-Head Neck Surg 2008;19(4):234–6.
44. Vairaktaris E, Vassiliou S, Yapijakis C, et al. Salivary Gland Manifestations of Sarcoidosis: Report of Three Cases. J Oral Maxillofacial Surg 2005;63(7): 1016–21.
45. Mansour MJ, He C, Al-Farra ST, et al. Sarcoidosis and Sjögren's syndrome: clinical and salivary evaluation. J Oral Pathol Med 2013;42(8):594–9.
46. Blaise P, Fardeau C, Chapelon C, et al. Minor salivary gland biopsy in diagnosing ocular sarcoidosis. Br J Ophthalmol 2011;95(12):1731–4.
47. Bernard C, Kodjikian L, Bancel B, et al. Ocular sarcoidosis: when should labial salivary gland biopsy be performed? Graefes Arch Clin Exp Ophthalmol 2013; 251(3):855–60.
48. Martín-Nares E, Ángeles-Ángeles A, Hernandez-Molina G. Major salivary gland enlargement in IgG4-related disease is associated with multiorgan involvement and higher basal disease activity. Mod Rheumatol 2020;30(1):172–7.
49. Karadeníz H, Vaglio A. IgG4-related disease: a contemporary review. Turk J Med Sci 2020;50(7):1616–31.

50. Puxeddu I, Capecchi R, Carta F, et al. Salivary Gland Pathology in IgG4-Related Disease: A Comprehensive Review. J Immunol Res 2018;2018:6936727.

51. Tachibana T, Orita Y, Wani Y, et al. Application of lip biopsy for the histological diagnosis of immunoglobulin G4-related disease. Ear Nose Throat J 2020. 145561320971932.

52. Sánchez Barrueco A, González Galán F, Alcalá Rueda I, et al. Incidence and risk factors for radioactive iodine-induced sialadenitis. Acta Otolaryngol 2020; 140(11):959–62.

53. Riachy R, Ghazal N, Haidar MB, et al. Early Sialadenitis After Radioactive Iodine Therapy for Differentiated Thyroid Cancer: Prevalence and Predictors. Int J Endocrinol 2020;2020:e8649794.

54. Kim YM, Choi JS, Hong SB, et al. Salivary gland function after sialendoscopy for treatment of chronic radioiodine-induced sialadenitis. Head & Neck 2016; 38(1):51–8.

55. Wu CB, Xi H, Zhou Q, et al. Sialendoscopy-Assisted Treatment for Radioiodine-Induced Sialadenitis. J Oral Maxillofacial Surg 2015;73(3):475–81.

56. Cung TD, Lai W, Svider PF, et al. Sialendoscopy in the Management of Radioiodine Induced Sialadenitis: A Systematic Review. Ann Otol Rhinol Laryngol 2017; 126(11):768–73.

57. Choi JS, Choi YG, Kim YM, et al. Clinical outcomes and prognostic factors of sialendoscopy in salivary duct stenosis. The Laryngoscope 2018;128(4):878–84.

58. Reed LF, Gillespie MB, Hackman T. Open Approaches to Stensen Duct Scar. Otolaryngologic Clin North Am 2021;54(3):521–30.

59. Goncalves M, Mantsopoulos K, Schapher M, et al. Ultrasound in the Assessment of Parotid Duct Stenosis. J Ultrasound Med 2019;38(11):2935–43.

60. Koch M, Iro H. Salivary duct stenosis: diagnosis and treatment. Acta Otorhinolaryngol Ital 2017;37(2):132–41.

61. Koch M, Zenk J, Iro H. Algorithms for Treatment of Salivary Gland Obstructions. Otolaryngologic Clin North Am 2009;42(6):1173–92.

62. Kandl JA, Ong AA, Gillespie MB. Pull-through sialodochoplasty for Stensen's megaduct. The Laryngoscope 2016;126(9):2003–5.

63. Jeon YT, Hong MP, Lee SJ, et al. Efficacy and safety of intraglandular botulinum toxin injections for treatment of sialadenosis. Clin Otolaryngol 2021;46(5):1131–5.

64. Ihrler S, Rath C, Zengel P, et al. Pathogenesis of sialadenosis: possible role of functionally deficient myoepithelial cells. Oral Surg Oral Med Oral Pathol Oral Radiol Endodontology 2010;110(2):218–23.

65. Colella G, Lo Giudice G, De Luca R, et al. Interventional sialendoscopy in parotidomegaly related to eating disorders. J Eat Disord 2021;9(1):25, sialendoscopy in parotidomegaly related to eating disorders.

66. Pape SA, MacLeod RI, McLean NR, et al. Sialadenosis of the salivary glands. Br J Plast Surg 1995;48(6):419–21.

67. Mashrah MA, Aldhohrah T, Abdelrehem A, et al. What is the best method for prevention of postparotidectomy Frey syndrome? Network meta-analysis. Head & Neck 2021;43(4):1345–58.

68. De Virgilio A, Costantino A, Russo E, et al. Different Surgical Strategies in the Prevention of Frey Syndrome: A Systematic Review and Meta-analysis. The Laryngoscope 2021;131(8):1761–8.

69. Marchese MR, Bussu F, Settimi S, et al. Not only gustatory sweating and flushing: Signs and symptoms associated to the Frey syndrome and the role of botulinum toxin A therapy. Head & Neck 2021;43(3):949–55.

70. Dai XM, Liu H, He J, et al. Treatment of postparotidectomy Frey syndrome with the interposition of temporalis fascia and sternocleidomastoid flaps. Oral Surg Oral Med Oral Pathol Oral Radiol 2015;119(5):514–21.

71. Melong JC, Rigby MH, Corsten M, et al. Prospective outcomes following drainless superficial parotidectomy with sternocleidomastoid flap reconstruction. J Otolaryngol - Head Neck Surg 2020;49(1):72.

The Online Physician Image
A Brave New World

Jordan P. Sand, MD, FACS[a,b,c],*

KEYWORDS

- Online reviews • Social media • Online reputation

KEY POINTS

- Internet searches and online reviews have become a ubiquitous part of the American experience.
- A plethora of online review sites exist for physicians, and patients are both reading these sites and providing content to these sites.
- Studies show that although the online reviews may not exactly correlate with the quality of care, patients are likely using these reviews to make decisions on which physicians to visit.
- Physicians should be aware of their online image and take measures to protect and direct their online reviews.

INTRODUCTION

When it comes to a physician's online image, there appear to be 3 attitudes that prevail:

1. Do not know about their online image, do not care to know about it.
2. Know about their online image, try not to care about it.
3. Know about their online image, make active effort to improve and refine.

Many physicians think that their online presence does not matter to patients as they have worked hard to secure their patient referrals and they know that they provide good medical care for their patients. They are board-certified and trained to provide top level care. These should be the qualifications that patients are looking for and they think it does not matter if they get positive or negative reviews from patients. Their practice is busy without investing effort in this portion of their business. Ultimately, the question is whether it is worth the effort to invest time and capital into ensuring that their online presence is positive. However, with the Internet becoming an integral part of our lives, the physician's online image is becoming more and more important

[a] Sand Plastic Surgery, 217 W Cataldo Avenue, Spokane, WA 99201, USA; [b] University of Washington School of Medicine, Seattle, WA, USA; [c] Washington State University School of Medicine
* Corresponding author. 217 W Cataldo Avenue, Spokane, WA 99201.
E-mail address: drsand@sandplasticsurgery.com

Surg Clin N Am 102 (2022) 233–239
https://doi.org/10.1016/j.suc.2021.12.003
0039-6109/22/© 2021 Elsevier Inc. All rights reserved.

to patients. Whether they should or not, patients do use reviews when they are researching their physician and will make medical care decisions with the information.

THE INTERNET CONNECTED WORLD

In this Internet-connected age, the first thing that many people do is go to an Internet search engine to discover answers to their questions. The framework built into the human consciousness is to research for health answers and typically Doctor Google is the first place that is queried. During the online search, the patient is bound to look up the physician who will be treating them. The first impression from the Internet search is important and lasting. Some patients will decide not to see a physician if they find something on their Internet search that causes them to be alarmed. Online reviews are used to make decisions, and this includes canceling an appointment or searching for another physician with a better online image. This can be particularly important for subspecialist physicians who receive referrals from other physicians for elective, outpatient procedures for which there is provider competition in the marketplace.

In addition, as cost sharing in most insurance plans has increased, patients have needed to become increasingly sensitive with the spending of health care dollars. Patients are often on high deductible plans and using their hard-earned money to pay for their medical care. When presented with an elective surgery, patients are willing to shop around to find the best provider for their procedure. Furthermore, as quality metrics have increasingly become tied to reimbursement, patient satisfaction is becoming a tracked value and being tied to reimbursement. Specifically, the HCAHPS survey of providers has been tied to reimbursement and several large national insurers are beginning to rate providers in their networks for their subscribers to find and identify. Notably, there are some types of work that are less elective or urgent/emergent, and so patient reviews or online presence is less of concern (ie, trauma surgery, on-call work, etc).

BUILDING A REPUTATION FOR REFERRALS

Historically, a subspecialist developed their reputation the "old-fashioned" way. They would move into a community and engage with the local physicians. As that occurred, word-of-mouth would spread among physicians and referrals began to build in the practice (based on medical skill, physician relationships, timeliness, communication, physician likability, etc). The referred patient would simply take the recommendation of their treating physician and did not look anywhere else. Additional word of mouth would spread within the community and many patients begin to self-refer. The physician's practice grows, and they often receive feedback from their patients in clinic, which enhances the physician's self-image. Although this was the method for building a practice for many years, the Internet and online reviews have changed this paradigm for patients.

In a study by Kinchen and colleagues, referring providers were asked what the most important aspects of choosing a specialist to send their patients.[1] The most important factor within the study was the medical skill of the individual who was taking the referral. This was a major factor for 87.5% of the survey respondents. The next most important factor was previous experience with the specialist, which was of major importance for 59.2% of the respondents. Other important factors included the appointment timeliness, quality of communication, likelihood of good patient-physician rapport, specialist returns to primary care, and insurance coverage. Less likely to be of importance was the fellowship training institution, medical school of graduation, that the specialist refers patients to the primary physician, office location, hospital affiliation, or attitudes of colleagues toward the specialist. The ability to get the job done is most important to the referring physician, which may not be a known reason to the patient who is being referred. Although a referring physician may not know or care about a subspecialist's online reviews, patients are likely looking up this information after being referred.

There has been extensive research into small businesses and online reviews, which likely partially extends to medical small businesses. In one study by inc.com, it was found that 91% of people regularly or occasionally read online reviews regarding a product or service.[2] Eighty-four percent of the respondents were likely to say that they trust the online reviews as much as a personal recommendation for the service. In addition, 68% are going to form their opinion after reading 1 to 6 reviews. Given that there is so much data available for individuals to sort through, a snap decision regarding a product or service is performed based on a cursory examination of reviews. A separate study from forbes.com had similar results, saying that 90% of individuals will decide based on online reviews.[3] Ninety-four percent of respondents will prefer a business with at least a 4-star rating. Importantly, 68% of respondents will leave a review if asked. Essentially, the results of these studies show that these reviews are used by individuals to make decisions and thus our email boxes are full of review requests from services that we use.

ONLINE REVIEWS IN MEDICINE

In the health care world, a multitude of review sites exists: Healthgrades.com, Vitals. com, Google.com, Yelp.com, RealSelf.com, GatherUp.com, Revolutionhealth.com, Facebook.com, WebMD.com, DrScore.com, Healthcarescoop.com, Nurses RecommendDoctors.com, RateMDs.com, ZocDoc.com, CareDash.com, Angie's List, Yahoo Local, Yellowpages.com, and so forth. These reviews usually come with star ratings with or without comments. According to healthgrades.com, half of all Americans who see a doctor each year will visit Healthgrades.com to look for information regarding their new physician or health care provider.[4] They also remark that there are at least 250 million visits to online physician review sites each year. The group Software Advice found that 77% of patients will use online reviews as their first step in finding a new physician.[5] They also found that almost half (47%) would go out-of-network to see a doctor with similar qualifications but had more favorable reviews. Meaning they are willing to pay a higher premium to see a higher-rated physician. In another study by Yaraghi and colleagues, when a patient was presented with a physician with a 4-star rating and a 2-star rating, the patient had a 31% higher chance of choosing the physician with the 4-star rating.[6]

Online reviews in medicine are also starting to get traction with insurance companies as they begin to use more data to help their enrolled customers choose within the network. Historically, Anthem Blue Cross Blue Shield has previously partnered with Zagat to help provide a forum for insurance members to review physicians.[7] There does appear to be a market desire for this information, as 51% of patients in one survey said that having public physician review comments were a good idea.[5] Physicians do seem to be adapting to the system, as in one study that showed 53% of providers look a review Web site and were likely to improve their own practices based on published patient experiences.[8] Although many studies do show some high level of importance to online reviews, one study from Mayo found that online reviews did not correlate with patient satisfaction survey responses.[9] This seems to demonstrate that online reviews are measuring something that may not exactly correlate with patient outcomes.

A different question is whether patients can recognize a poorly performing provider and online reviews reflect that a provider gave a substandard level of care. In one review by Murphy and colleagues, they found that Web reviews were lower for physicians who were on probation for their medical license, and it may be that patients can perceive a substandard level of care.[10] A separate study looked at "America's Top Doctor" to see if physicians reviewing physicians could pick up on a physician who provided substandard care. In the study by McGrath et al., no differences were found overall between online patient ratings and physician peer review status (America's Top Doctor).[11] There were, however, some statistical differences within 4 specialties (family medicine, allergists, internal medicine, and pediatrics) where online patient ratings were significantly higher for those physicians listed as peer-reviewed "Top Doctor" versus those who were not.

Further studies have been more critical of online patient reviews. In a study by Daskivich and colleagues, online physician ratings failed to predict actual performance on measures of quality, value, and peer review.[12] This study reviewed 78 physicians across 8 specialties and compared patient online review scores with quality metrics. Overall, they found that online reviews of specialist physicians did not predict objective measures of quality of care or peer assessment of clinical performance. This study group found that online patient review scores of individual physicians are consistent across platforms, suggesting that reviews jointly measure a latent construct that is unrelated to classically measured medical performance categories.

Some online review study has been done in the field of Otolaryngology by Sobin and colleagues.[13] A total of 281 faculty members in 25 programs were studied for review profiles on Vitals (70%) and Healthgrades (82%). They found that 49 identified comments (27%) were negative, and 138 otolaryngologists (49%) had at least 1 negative comment. They did find that academic position and subspecialty appeared to correlate with reviews ratings on Healthgrades. However, the state of practice and number of years in practice did not influence the reviews. They also found that facial plastic surgeons specifically had the lowest ratings in the study.

WHAT IS A REVIEW WORTH?

Although patients do seem to be looking and leaving reviews, the question becomes what a good or bad review is worth. Realself.com claims that a single good review is worth more than $1000 in marketing value.[14] An additional survey study has found that 50% of customers will pay more or travel further to utilized businesses with top reviews.[15] Seventy-two percent will trust a local business more because of positive reviews and 72% will act after reading one positive review. Reviews create action in individuals that this may mean more consults and more business. Negative reviews have a profound effect as well. In one study, they found that bad reviews in a google search can cause 70% of viewers to turn away.[16] However, responding to the bad review can lead to 70% of consumers returning to the business. A business with 4 negative reviews can risk up to 70% of people looking at the site to opt not to come to that site of business.[17]

As these reviews have become more prevalent and the data demonstrating that they have a major impact on consumer decisions, health care providers are taking more action against negative reviews. There are numerous cases of hospitals and physicians suing online review sites and patients to have the content removed that is felt to be false or derogatory. As review sites have legal protection from the content posted on their platforms, the hospital system or physician must sue the patient to have the review removed. There have been multiple successful lawsuits against libelous reviews. One case was brought by a Cleveland Clinic Urologist against a patient who posted negative comments about him for 10 years online. This case was settled with a settlement paid by the patient. A $12M judgment was awarded to Desert Palm Plastic surgery against a jazz singer who stated that she had a botched rhinoplasty performed by the group. Other surgeons and hospital groups have active lawsuits which are in the news regarding the removal of negative reviews from their online presence. This is a risky and expensive method to have the review removed from your online profile.

Notably, patients are instructed to look at online reviews when they are making care decisions. When searching for a physician, the popular media site US News instructs prospective patients to look for ranking lists, family and friend recommendations, on-line bios, and reviews.[17] In this guide, they also provide a caveat regarding online reviews, saying that opinions posted online should be taken with a grain of salt. Although these online guides to help patients find their physician take online reviews seriously, the author believes that the physician whose profile is linked to the online reviews should also take them seriously.

TODAY'S ONLINE PHYSICIAN IMAGE

As information gathering has evolved, so has the specialist focus on the online image as well. Although the physicians of the past relied on word of mouth to help grow their practice, the physician of the now will use the Internet to help grow their practice rapidly. Typically, when a specialist sets up a practice, they will pay for search engine optimization and a social media presence to get the word out. They will focus on asking their patients to leave online reviews to help build their online presence. When patients perform Web searches about their symptoms or for their physician, they will be overwhelmed with the positive reviews and top search hits for the special-ist's Web site and will set up an appointment post-haste.

Although the online review content has grown, so has the gaming of the content by physicians as well. This has created several ethical questions regarding online review and physician professionalism. Is it ethical to maintain your own review site? Is it ethical to ask patients for reviews knowing the physician will sway toward those who are going to leave a positive review? Is it ethical to pay a patient to perform a re-view? Is it ethical to sue a patient for a review? Is it ethical to have fake reviews (either positive or negative)? Many of these questions seem to have obvious answers, but sit-uations may vary, and each scenario would be judged on the individual circumstances.

SUMMARY

In summary, online reviews are ubiquitous and patients use this information to make decisions regarding their health care. Although some studies demonstrate that these reviews do not appear to correlate with standard metrics of patient care, there is some correlation with a substandard care delivery by a practitioner. There is a latent metric that is being defined in online physician reviews, and it is unclear if this has a major impact on patient outcomes. However, although the evidence of what a patient might do with a physician's online review is conflicting, many studies seem to identify that these reviews are being taken at face value. In addition, the fact that many lawsuits have been filed to remove reviews means that practices are taking these reviews very seriously. Additional research is, however, needed to identify how online reviews impact the patient choice of a physician.

With this information, how should a physician approach their online image? This author believes that with the omnipresent nature of online reviews, it is too late for a physician to ignore their online presence and let it play out without any intervention. A physician must confront their online presence and work to take control of the information being presented. A provider should ask their patients to leave reviews and focus one's efforts to build up a positive online presence. A provider should google their name or clinic at least once per quarter to see what is being said about them online. They should read and respond to the reviews that are on their various profiles. They should be aware of what potential patients are reading about them before their office visits. An opinion about the provider will often be formed before the patient is even seen. The best way to drown out a negative review is to have copious positive reviews. One should take their own reviews with a grain of salt as often the most motived patients to write reviews are upset. To help solicit reviews, a practice may create a card to hand to patients to help elicit positive reviews. Practices should aim to request patients to cross-post to several different platforms to help build the online profile. Alternatively, the practice can hire a service to help accomplish this and automate review requests. Many of these types of companies exist. Although patient reviews of physicians may be perceived as fatuous by physicians, the content is rapidly growing and available to patients. This author believes that a practice or physician must have a plan to address it.

CLINICS CARE POINTS

- Online physician image is evolving to become an important part of a medical practice.
- While online reviews may not directly correlate with clinical care quality studied by other metrics, patients continue to utilize this information for medical care decitions.

DISCLOSURE

The author has nothing to disclose.

REFERENCES

1. Kinchen KS, Cooper LA, Levine D, et al. Referral of patients to specialists: factors affecting choice of specialist by primary care physicians. Ann Fam Med 2004; 2(3):245–52.
2. Bloem C. (2021, September 14) 84 percent of people trust online reviews as much as friends. Here's how to manage what they see. Available at: https://www.inc.com/craig-bloem/84-percent-of-people-trust-online-reviews-as-much-.htm. Accessed October 1, 2021.
3. Capoccia C. (2018, April 11) online reviews are the best thing that ever happened to small business. Available at: https://www.forbes.com/sites/forbestechcouncil/2018/04/11/online-reviews-are-the-best-thing-that-ever-happened-to-small-businesses/#5b1c406740a0. Accessed October 1, 2021.
4. Healthgrades Marketplace, LLC. 2021. Available at: http://www.healthgrades.com. Accessed October 1, 2021.
5. Hedges L, Collin C. (2020, April 3) How patients use online reviews. Available at: https://www.softwareadvice.com/resources/how-patients-use-online-reviews/. Accessed October 1, 2021.
6. Yaraghi N, Wang W, Gao GG, et al. How online quality ratings influence patients' choice of medical providers: controlled experimental survey Study. J Med Internet Res 2018;20(3):e99.

7. Pasternak A, Scherger JE. Online reviews of physicians: what are your patients posting about you? Fam Pract Manag 2009;16(3):9–11.
8. Heath S. (2017, February 6) Online physician reviews stressful for docs, useful for patients. Available at: https://patientengagementhit.com/news/online-physician-reviews-stressful-for-docs-useful-for-patients. Accessed October 1, 2021.
9. Widmer RJ, Maurer MJ, Nayar VR, et al. Online physician reviews do not reflect patient satisfaction survey responses. Mayo Clin Proc 2018;93(4):453–7.
10. Murphy GP, Awad MA, Osterberg EC, et al. Web-based physician ratings for california physicians on probation. J Med Internet Res 2017;19(8):e254.
11. McGrath RJ, Priestley JL, Zhou Y, et al. The validity of online patient ratings of physicians: analysis of physician peer reviews and patient ratings. Interact J Med Res 2018;7(1):e8.
12. Daskivich TJ, Houman J, Fuller G, et al. Online physician ratings fail to predict actual performance on measures of quality, value, and peer review. J Am Med Inform Assoc 2018;25(4):401–7.
13. Sobin L, Goyal P. Trends of online ratings of otolaryngologists: what do your patients really think of you? JAMA Otolaryngol Head Neck Surg 2014;140(7):635–8.
14. Realself, Inc.. 2021. Available at: http://www.realself.com. Accessed October 1, 2021.
15. Podium Corp Inc. (2021) 2021 State of Online Reviews. Available at: https://www.podium.com/state-of-online-reviews/. Accessed October 1, 2021.
16. Quora Inc. (2021). Available at: https://www.quora.com/How-much-does-a-bad-review-cost-your-business-Are-there-any-studies-that-can-help-me-prove-that-bad-reviews-will-hurt-my-client's-sales-and-revenue.
17. Howley EK. How to find a good doctor. 2020. Available at: https://health.usnews.com/health-care/patient-advice/articles/2018-01-09/how-to-find-the-best-primary-care-doctor. Accessed October 1, 2021.

Head and Neck Radiation Therapy
From Consultation to Survivorship and Future Directions

Zachary David Guss, MD, MSc

KEYWORDS

- Radiation oncology • Radiation • Toxicity • Head and neck

KEY POINTS

- Radiation therapy is a key component of therapy for many patients who receive treatment for head and neck cancer.
- Advanced radiation oncology techniques ensure comprehensive and safe treatment.
- Continuing efforts aim to improve the effectiveness and decrease the toxicity of radiation oncology for head and neck cancer.

BACKGROUND

Radiation oncology, along with head and neck surgery and medical oncology, constitutes one of the central pillars of care for head and neck cancers. This article will review the essential components of a patient's journey through radiation oncology. Future directions and areas of research are also discussed.

INITIAL CONSULTATION

When a patient is referred to a radiation oncologist for a new diagnosis of head and neck cancer, a clinic visit is arranged. After a complete history and physical examination (and nasopharyngolaryngoscopy as appropriate), the radiation oncologist will review the treatment options and their associated side effects. Close communication among the head and neck surgeon, radiation oncologist, and medical oncologist (as applicable) is essential. For postoperative cases, discussions between the head and neck surgeon and radiation oncologist can reveal insights and nuances beyond what is evident from the pathology report. Typically, external beam radiation therapy is performed for head and neck cancers. In external beam radiation therapy, the most common technique is to use a linear accelerator (LINAC) to generate high-energy

Deaconess Hospital Radiation Oncology, MultiCare Health System, 910 W 5th Avenue, Suite 102b, Spokane, WA 99204, USA
E-mail address: Zach0001@multicare.org

Surg Clin N Am 102 (2022) 241–249
https://doi.org/10.1016/j.suc.2021.12.004

photons (x-rays) that are aimed at tumors or areas at risk of subclinical involvement. Although there are many nuances and exceptions, patients treated with curative intent generally receive 7 weeks (70 Gray [Gy—the unit of measurement for radiation dose]) of radiation therapy delivered 5 times weekly for intact tumors or 60 to 66 Gy delivered over 6 to 6.5 weeks, 5 times weekly, in the postoperative setting.[1] If radiation therapy is recommended and the patient would like to proceed with treatment, informed consent is obtained. The patient will then be scheduled for a computed tomography (CT) based radiation therapy simulation, which functions as the planning session. Referrals to allied fields such as nutrition, speech-language pathology (for swallow therapy), audiology, and dentistry are often placed at the time of consultation.

SIMULATION

The radiation therapy simulation consists of a CT scan, with or without contrast, that generates a 3-dimensional image of a patient's anatomy. These images form the basis upon which target delineation is constructed, as well as identification of areas of risk, during the radiation therapy planning process. Hence, devices must be used to ensure that the patient's positioning at the time of simulation can be reproduced each day throughout the 6- to 7-week course of radiation therapy. For head and neck cancer, immobilization usually requires the creation of a custom thermoplastic mask. It is at first soft, wet, and warm, and it is stretched over the patient's face, neck, and shoulders. As it dries, the plastic hardens.

In addition to the mask, additional devices and techniques can be used to maximize clinical outcomes. There are a variety of mouthpieces and tongue depressors that can be used in select circumstances to reproducibly displace uninvolved portions of the oral cavity from the high-dose target region.[2,3]

In the postoperative setting, radiopaque adhesive wires are generally placed along surgical scars to maximize visibility on CT imaging. Additional material can be placed along surgical scars, particularly if there was extranodal extension on final pathology, to increase skin dose in designated regions.

TREATMENT PLANNING

The CT images obtained during the simulation are sent to a radiation oncology software program for contouring targets and organs at risk (OARs). Often, additional diagnostic studies are needed for the accurate delineation of these regions. For head and neck radiation therapy, diagnostic PET/CTs, contrast-enhanced CTs (if contrast was not administered during the radiation therapy simulation), and MRI can assist the radiation oncologist. For postoperative cases, importing both preoperative and postoperative diagnostic scans is helpful. These images can be overlaid on the simulation CT to provide additional insights into locations where gross and microscopic disease may be located.

Owing to differences in positioning, weight change, and anatomic change (for postoperative patients), performing a "rigid" registration in the diagnostic scan in which voxels are matched 1:1 between the simulation CT and diagnostic imaging can mislead the radiation oncologist's interpretation of where cancer may be located. For head and neck radiation therapy, it is often preferable to perform a "deformable" registration that can help account for anatomic change to more accurately (if performed properly) determine areas at risk.

After the image registrations have been performed, OARs that need to be protected and targets that require radiation are identified on the simulation CT through the process of contouring. There can be significant variation in radiation target delineation among radiation oncologists. In recent years, several resources including consensus guidelines and online modules have emerged to standardize approaches.[4–6] Head and neck contouring is generally perceived to be challenging and nuanced. Intensive peer review of physician contours has been implemented in many centers to improve quality.[7–9]

A full discussion of contouring practices across head and neck subsites is beyond the scope of this article. Here, several key concepts are reviewed. If there is visible tumor by physical examination or imaging in the primary site and/or neck, a gross tumor volume (GTV) is contoured. Dependent on the primary site and histopathologic features (eg, perineural invasion), areas at risk for harboring microscopic disease are contoured as the clinical target volume (CTV). The CTV can consist of a set margin applied to the GTV while respecting anatomic barriers to tumor spread or elective coverage of head and neck lymph node groups and cranial nerves. Furthermore, CTVs may be categorized into different dose levels dependent on the perceived risk. For example, a patient with oral cavity cancer who underwent resection of the primary and neck would have a higher dose prescribed to the CTV for a cervical lymph node level that harbored a lymph node with extranodal extension compared with a different level on the same side of the neck that harbored noninvolved lymph nodes. Finally, planning target volumes (PTVs) are constructed by performing a geometric expansion around the CTVs. The PTV is typically a few millimeters and accounts for uncertainty and slight variations that may occur day to day in alignment.

Although there are many different approaches, one common dose scheme for definitive cases comprises prescribing 70 Gy to the high-risk CTV, 63 Gy to the intermediate-risk CTV, and 56 Gy to the low-risk CTV, in 35 daily treatments (fractions). Thus, each day, the various targets will receive a slightly different dose of radiation. Varying dose allows the radiation oncologist to prioritize areas dependent on their perceived risk to the patient and spare toxicity where the highest doses are not felt to be necessary.

Head and neck cancer radiation therapy treatment would be straightforward if the only objective was to treat areas at risk to the dose required to eradicate the tumor cells. However, the head and neck comprises dozens of anatomic structures that must be protected. Many have a maximum dose tolerance below that of the dose required for the PTVs. Therefore, OARs such as the brainstem, spinal cord, major salivary glands, mandible, and optic structures must also be contoured. The "art of medicine" lies in treating the tumor adequately while minimizing the risk of harm to the patient.

To achieve this aim, radiation oncologists work in close collaboration with dosimetrists, who are highly trained analytical members of the team who specialize in treatment planning. The radiation oncologist provides plan objectives to the dosimetrist, who enters this information into the treatment planning software. Most cases are too complex for forward planning, in which the dosimetrist places beams of radiation therapy upfront to treat the targets delineated by the radiation oncologist. Instead, most head and neck plans use inverse planning, in which the objectives that a physician desires (eg, "make sure all of the GTV receives 70 Gy but also do not let the spinal cord maximum dose reach over 45 Gy") are used by computer algorithms to generate radiation therapy plans that best satisfy these objectives. There are often many objectives, sometimes in conflict, and they are often weighted by importance to the physician. The physician and dosimetrist then review the best plans, revise objectives in case the plans are unacceptable, and ultimately select the best plan. The treatment planning systems have grown more sophisticated to match the evolution of the LINACs. For example, the treatment planning system can devise a plan in which the

LINAC head rotates around the patient while tungsten leaves within the head form intricate patterns to create highly conformal plans in which the dose falls off sharply beyond the edge of the PTV. After a plan is approved, additional quality assurance and safety checks are performed by the dosimetrist, physicist, and radiation therapist to ensure that the plan can be safely delivered to the patient.

TREATMENT DELIVERY

Radiation therapy for curative-intent treatment of head and neck cancers is typically delivered over 6 to 7 weeks, 5 days per week. Each day, the patient is positioned on the LINAC by radiation therapists, the mask is placed over the patient and fastened to the treatment table, and a low-dose cone-beam CT (CBCT) scan without contrast is obtained. The therapists will compare the CBCT to the planning CT to determine whether any adjustments in patient position are necessary. When alignment is satisfactory, treatment is delivered. Treatments are generally delivered quickly once the patient is positioned properly, and patients can expect to spend approximately 20 minutes in the department each day. The radiation oncologist reviews the CBCT before the next treatment is delivered to ensure proper patient alignment. High-quality image guidance requires not only that the patient is being positioned properly by the radiation therapist team but also that weight loss and tumor response are not so significant as to demand repeat simulation and replanning. A representative case demonstrating contouring, radiation planning, and image guidance is provided in **Fig. 1**.

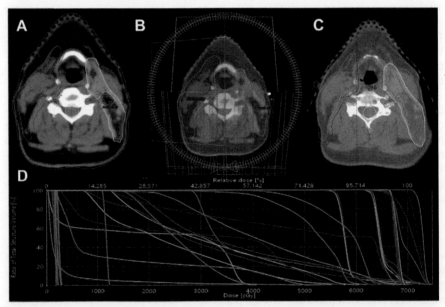

Fig. 1. (A) After the CT-based radiation therapy planning session (simulation), the targets and OARs are contoured. (B) Colorwash representation of the dose distribution depicting different levels of risk receiving different levels of dose. The right side of the neck is redder and receives a higher dose, whereas the spinal cord receives a much lower dose in this plan. (C) CBCT from the patient's daily treatment imaging demonstrating alignment of the patient with the overlaid contours from the planning session. (D) Dose-volume histogram for this patient's plan, depicting dose distributions for the targets and OARs. This is one of several tools that ensures a proper balance of aggressiveness toward the cancer while respecting normal tissue constraints.

ON TREATMENT MANAGEMENT

Radiation therapy patients are generally seen by the radiation oncologist once each week. In this visit, the radiation oncologist assesses and manages toxicity and reviews laboratories and other diagnostic tests. The anticipated morbidity of head and neck radiation therapy treatment course is dependent on multiple factors including the anatomic subsite of the primary, the technical aspects of the radiation therapy plan, the patient's performance status and comorbidities, and the presence or absence of concurrent systemic therapy. Common acute toxicities include mucositis, dermatitis, and pain. Supportive medications include topical skincare products, viscous lidocaine, and opioid analgesics. Doxepin and gabapentin have been studied to reduce the burden of symptomatic oral mucositis.[10–12] The patient's weight must be watched closely; if caloric demands are not being met, a gastrostomy tube may be necessary.

FOLLOW-UP AND SURVIVORSHIP

Patients with head and neck cancer typically undergo a thorough re-evaluation 3 months after the completion of radiation therapy to assess tumor response and manage toxicity. In the definitive setting, initial follow-up often comprises a detailed history and physical examination, PET/CT, and nasopharyngolaryngoscopy to document a complete response to treatment. If the response is favorable, then the radiation oncologist and head and neck surgeon monitor the patient for recurrence at initially short intervals that lengthen as the time goes on. If recurrence arises, salvage treatments can be considered.

In addition to surveillance, the radiation oncologist must address survivorship and the management of late effects. Swallowing dysfunction, xerostomia, fibrosis of the irradiated tissues, hypothyroidism, and chronic pain are among the potential late effects of head and neck radiation therapy. Smoking cessation counseling is frequently indicated as it has been tied to oncologic outcomes.[13]

FUTURE DIRECTIONS

Researchers are working hard to improve the oncologic outcomes, toxicity profiles, and convenience of head and neck radiation therapy. A selection of promising strategies is reviewed in this section.

IMPROVING ONCOLOGIC OUTCOMES

For patients with unfavorable head and neck cancer, trials are testing the role of checkpoint inhibitor immunotherapy. The clinical trial NRG-HN003 is evaluating the addition of pembrolizumab to standard of care chemoradiation in patients with high-risk head and neck cancer who face poor prognosis with today's standard regimens. Treatment intensification in this manner may lead to improved outcomes.[14]

There are patients who cannot receive cisplatin because of various comorbidities. These patients often receive concurrent cetuximab. Cetuximab is an EGFR binding monoclonal antibody that has been demonstrated to be superior to radiation alone for locoregionally advanced head and neck cancer but inferior to concurrent cisplatin.[15,16] The clinical trial NRG-HN004 aims to improve oncologic outcomes for this group of patients by testing whether the checkpoint inhibitor durvalumab is better than cetuximab.[17]

Treatment can also be intensified by increasing the dose of radiation delivered each day. For example, the Dose-Escalated Hypofractionated Adaptive Radiotherapy for Head and Neck Cancer (DEHART) trial aims to deliver up to double the dose of daily radiation therapy over only 15 days of treatment with combined atezolizumab checkpoint inhibitor.[18] This trial also uses a new LINAC modality with MRI guidance rather than standard CT-guided radiation therapy to make changes to the radiation therapy plan during therapy as indicated by tumor response in real time.

REDUCING TOXICITY

Fortunately, many head and neck cancers can be cured with single or combined modality approaches involving surgery, radiation therapy, and chemotherapy. For patients with a favorable prognosis, such as human papillomavirus (HPV)-associated squamous cell carcinoma of the oropharynx, research has been focused on de-escalating therapy without compromising historically high cure rates. There are many ways to reduce toxicity, and this review highlights the following 3 approaches: reducing radiation dose, adding radioprotectors, and reducing the size of the radiation target.

With respect to radiation dose reduction, most efforts have centered on HPV-associated oropharynx cancer. The clinical trial NRG-HN002 recently reported findings of the phase II component of the study evaluating reduced dose (60 Gy over 6 weeks vs the standard 70 Gy over 7 weeks) radiation therapy with or without concurrent cisplatin.[19] The arm with concurrent chemotherapy met its prespecified endpoint and will advance to a phase III trial. NRG-HN005 is a multi-institutional phase II/III study that seeks to determine the impact of both reducing radiation dose and substituting the checkpoint nivolumab for cisplatin in a 3-arm design.[20] Another avenue to reduce dose is to combine surgery with a reduced postoperative radiation dose. ECOG-ACRIN 3311 aimed to evaluate the role of transoral robotic surgical resection followed by randomization to low- or standard-dose IMRT in resectable p16+ oropharynx cancer. In this phase II study, patients with low-risk disease appeared to fare well with transoral surgery followed by 50 Gy, which is 10 Gy below current standard of care dosing.[21] However, it must be noted that a reduction in radiation dose in this manner comes at the cost of introducing surgical toxicity. For example, the ORATOR phase II randomized trial demonstrated similar swallowing function with transoral robotic surgery followed by risk-adapted (based on pathology) postoperative radiation therapy or chemoradiation compared to definitive radiation therapy or chemoradiation.[22]

Radioprotectors represent an additional avenue to spare toxicity. To be useful in the clinic, the agent must protect normal tissues more than it protects tumor cells. A phase IIb randomized, double-blind trial of GC4419 versus placebo to reduce oral mucositis due to concurrent radiotherapy and cisplatin for head and neck cancer demonstrated a reduction of symptomatic oral mucositis with respect to symptom duration, incidence, and severity.[23] This is currently being studied in the phase III ROMAN: A Study to Investigate the Effects of GC4419 on Radiation Induced Oral Mucositis in Patients With Head/Neck Cancer clinical trial.[24]

Another way to reduce toxicity is to reduce the amount of tissue receiving radiation. Rather than reduce the dose, the size of the various dose targets is simply reduced, and the uninvolved but proximal normal tissues thus receive a lower dose. One way to accomplish this is to use knowledge of patterns of spread to remove elective nodal coverage that harbors a low risk of carrying occult disease. Memorial Sloan-Kettering has published its approach to reducing the target size and dose of elective neck radiation while maintaining standard of care radiation dose to the target in HPV-associated squamous cell carcinoma of the oropharynx patients who receive concurrent cisplatin.[25] Excellent short-term locoregional control rates have been reported. An alternative is to use a different form of radiation therapy called proton therapy to reduce the dose to nearby OARs. A discussion of the benefits and drawbacks of proton therapy versus standard high-energy x-ray (photon) radiation is beyond the scope of the article, but in general, proton therapy can cover the radiation target with a sharper dose fall off.[26] In a treatment planning system, the proton plans will generally look favorable. However, the high-dose region remains similar, and there are no randomized comparative data demonstrating that toxicity profiles are improved with this technology. It is important to conduct such research given proton therapy's limited availability and increased cost. Fortunately, this is now being studied in a prospective clinical trial.[27]

SUMMARY

Radiation therapy is an important component of care for many patients with head and neck cancer. From initial consultation through treatment planning and delivery, multidisciplinary discussion with head and neck surgery and medical oncology is critical to ensure best outcomes. Although sophisticated methods are already in place to maximize benefits and minimize harm, head and neck radiation can have significant acute and late effects. Ongoing research efforts aim to improve cure rates and reduce toxicity.

DISCLOSURE

The author has nothing to disclose.

REFERENCES

1. Head and Neck Cancers Version 3.2021. 2021. Available at: https://www.nccn. org/professionals/physician_gls/pdf/head-and-neck.pdfhttps://www.nccn.org/ professionals/physician_gls/pdf/head-and-neck.pdf. Accessed January 1, 2022.

2. Precise Bite Patient Re-Positioner. Precise bite patient re-positioner. (n.d.). Available at: https://civcort.com/ro/head-neck/precise-bite/Precise-Bite-Patient-Re-Positioner.htm. Accessed January 1, 2022.

3. Stieb S, Perez-Martinez I, Mohamed ASR, et al. The impact of tongue-deviating and tongue-depressing oral stents on long-term radiation-associated symptoms in oropharyngeal cancer survivors. Clin translational Radiat Oncol 2020;24:71–8.

4. Grégoire V, Evans M, Le QT, et al. Delineation of the primary tumour Clinical Target Volumes (CTV-P) in laryngeal, hypopharyngeal, oropharyngeal and oral cavity squamous cell carcinoma: AIRO, CACA, DAHANCA, EORTC, GEORCC, GORTEC, HKNPCSG, HNCIG, IAG-KHT, LPRHHT, NCIC CTG, NCRI, NRG Oncology, PHNS, SBRT, SOMERA, SRO, SSHNO, TROG consensus guidelines. Radiotherapy and oncology. J Eur Soc Ther Radiol Oncol 2018;126(1):3–24.

5. Lee AW, Ng WT, Pan JJ, et al. International guideline for the delineation of the clinical target volumes (CTV) for nasopharyngeal carcinoma. Radiother Oncol 2018; 126(1):25–36.

6. Tata Medical Center RSNA AVARO anatomy project. econtour.org. (n.d.). Available at: https://www.econtour.org/cases/83. Accessed January 1, 2022.

7. Ramasamy S, Murray LJ, Cardale K, et al. Quality assurance peer review of head and neck contours in a large cancer centre via a weekly meeting approach. Clin Oncol (Royal Coll Radiol) 2019;31(6):344–51.

8. Fong C, Sanghera P, Good J, et al. Implementing head and neck contouring peer review without pathway delay: the on-demand approach. Clin Oncol (R Coll Radiol) 2017;29(12):841–7.

9. Zairis S, Margalit DN, Royce TJ, et al. Prospective analysis of radiation oncology image and plan-driven peer review for head and neck cancer. Head Neck 2017; 39(8):1603–8.

10. Bar Ad V, Weinstein G, Dutta PR, et al. Gabapentin for the treatment of pain related to radiation-induced mucositis in patients with head and neck tumors treated with intensity-modulated radiation therapy. Head Neck 2010;32(2):173–7.

11. Milazzo-Kiedaisch CA, Itano J, Dutta PR. Role of gabapentin in managing mucositis pain in patients undergoing radiation therapy to the head and neck. Clin J Oncol Nurs 2016;20(6):623–8.

12. Jayakrishnan R, Chang K, Ugurluer G, et al. Doxepin for radiation therapy-induced mucositis pain in the treatment of oral cancers. Oncol Rev 2015; 9(1):290.

13. van Imhoff LC, Kranenburg GG, Macco S, Nijman NL, van Overbeeke EJ, Wegner I,, Pothen AJ. Prognostic value of continued smoking on survival and recurrence rates in patients with head and neck cancer: A systematic review. Head & neck 2016;38(Suppl 1):E2214–20.

14. NRG-HN003 Cisplatin, Intensity-Modulated radiation therapy, and Pembrolizumab in treating patients with stage III-IV head and neck squamous cell carcinoma. 2018. Available at: https://clinicaltrials.gov/ct2/show/NCT02775812. Accessed January 1, 2022.

15. Bonner JA, Harari PM, Giralt J, et al. Radiotherapy plus cetuximab for squamous-cell carcinoma of the head and neck. N Engl J Med 2006;354(6):567–78.

16. Gillison ML, Trotti AM, Harris J, et al. Radiotherapy plus cetuximab or cisplatin in human papillomavirus-positive oropharyngeal cancer (NRG Oncology RTOG 1016): a randomised, multicentre, non-inferiority trial. Lancet 2019;393(10166): 40–50.

17. Radiation therapy with durvalumab or cetuximab in treating patients with locoregionally advanced head and neck cancer who cannot Take Cisplatin. 2017. Available at: https://clinicaltrials.gov/ct2/show/NCT03258554. Accessed January 1, 2022.

18. Dose-Escalated Hypofractionated Adaptive Radiotherapy for head and neck cancer. 2020. Available at: https://clinicaltrials.gov/ct2/show/NCT04477759. Accessed January 1, 2022.

19. Yom SS, Torres-Saavedra P, Caudell JJ, et al. Reduced-Dose Radiation Therapy for HPV-Associated Oropharyngeal Carcinoma (NRG Oncology HN002). J Clin Oncol 2021;39(9):956–65.

20. De-intensified radiation therapy with CHEMOTHERAPY (Cisplatin) or IMMUNO-THERAPY (NIVOLUMAB) in treating patients With Early-Stage, HPV-Positive, Non-Smoking Associated Oropharyngeal cancer. 2019. Available at: https://clinicaltrials.gov/ct2/show/NCT03952585. Accessed January 1, 2022.

21. Ferris RL, Flamand Y, Weinstein GS, et al. Transoral robotic surgical resection followed by randomization to low- or standard-dose IMRT in resectable p16+ locally advanced oropharynx cancer: A trial of the ECOG-ACRIN Cancer Research Group (E3311). J Clin Oncol 2020;38(15_suppl):6500.

22. Nichols AC, Theurer J, Prisman E, Read N, Berthelet E, Tran E,, Palma DA. Radiotherapy versus transoral robotic surgery and neck dissection for oropharyngeal squamous cell carcinoma (ORATOR): an open-label, phase 2, randomised trial. Lancet Oncol 2019;20(10):1349–59.

23. Anderson CM, Lee CM, Saunders DP, et al. Phase IIb, Randomized, Double-Blind Trial of GC4419 versus placebo to reduce severe oral mucositis due to concurrent radiotherapy and cisplatin for head and neck cancer. J Clin Oncol 2019; 37(34):3256–65.
24. Roman: A study to investigate the effects of gc4419 on radiation induced oral mucositis in patients with head/neck cancer. 2018. Available at: https://clinicaltrials.gov/ct2/show/NCT03689712. Accessed January 1, 2022.
25. Tsai CJ, McBride SM, Riaz N, et al. Reducing the Radiation Therapy Dose Prescription for Elective Treatment Areas in Human Papillomavirus-Associated Oropharyngeal Carcinoma Being Treated With Primary Chemoradiotherapy at Memorial Sloan Kettering Cancer Center. Pract Radiat Oncol 2019;9(2):98–101.
26. Håkansson K, Smulders B, Specht L, et al. Radiation dose-painting with protons vs. photons for head-and-neck cancer. Acta Oncol 2020;59(5):525–33.
27. Study of proton versus photon beam radiotherapy in the treatment of head and neck cancer. 2016. Available at: https://clinicaltrials.gov/ct2/show/NCT02923570.

Contemporary Management of Primary Hyperparathyroidism

Lauren Slattery, MD[a], Jason P. Hunt, MD[b],*

KEYWORDS

- Primary hyperparathyroidism • Minimally invasive • Localization

KEY POINTS

- Primary hyperparathyroidism can be asymptomatic or symptomatic, as well as classic, normocalcemic, or normohormonal.
- Preoperative localization with imaging is necessary for a minimally invasive approach and can be helpful even if planning 4-gland exploration.
- There are a variety of intraoperative techniques that can be helpful including intraoperative PTH monitoring, radioguidance, venous sampling, and fluorescence techniques, among others.

INTRODUCTION

Primary hyperparathyroidism (PHPT) is a common disorder that affects women more than men with an incidence of 66 per 100,000 person-years in women versus 25 per 100,000 person-years in men.[1] The autonomous secretion of parathyroid hormone (PTH) typically leads to elevation of serum calcium and reduction of phosphorus levels. However, there are variations in clinical presentation that must be considered.

PHPT can cause a multitude of adverse effects for an individual including bone disease, musculoskeletal discomfort, nephrolithiasis, gastrointestinal disease, and neuropsychiatric disease, among others. This can affect quality of life in the short term, whereas the long-term effects are typically much more clinically significant and most commonly include osteoporosis and renal disease, as well as potential effects on blood pressure and heart disease.[2–4] In addition to preventing end-organ damage, parathyroidectomy can improve anxiety, depression, cognitive dysfunction, constipation, and nausea, which have also been linked to prolonged hypercalcemia.[5]

Management is tailored to the individual and includes observation, medical management, or surgical/procedural management. In recent years, technological advances have improved localization of disease. However, the primary management

[a] University of Utah, 50 N Medical Drive, Salt Lake City, UT 84132, USA; [b] University of Utah, Huntsman Cancer Institute, 50 N Medical Drive, 3C120SOM, Salt Lake City, UT 84132, USA
* Corresponding author.
E-mail address: jason.hunt@hsc.utah.edu

Surg Clin N Am 102 (2022) 251–265
https://doi.org/10.1016/j.suc.2021.12.009
0039-6109/22/© 2022 Elsevier Inc. All rights reserved.

surgical.theclinics.com

remains surgical with parathyroidectomy being the standard of care. Surgery is curative in approximately 97% to 98% of cases.[6–8] During workup and in surgery, the surgeon needs to be prepared for multiple possibilities of involved glands. In approximately 80% to 90% cases, there is a single adenoma that is encountered.[6] In addition, multiple adenomas are encountered in approximately 1% to 10% and 4-gland hyperplasia in 1% to 20% of cases.[6,9,10]

This review focuses on the diagnosis, localization, surgical management, and alternatives to surgical management of PHPT.

WORKUP AND CLINICAL CONSIDERATIONS

A common presentation of hyperparathyroidism is incidentally noted hypercalcemia. Subtle hypercalcemia on laboratory evaluation has the potential to be ignored by practitioners unless associated with end-organ damage or symptomatic events such as recurrent kidney stones. Hypercalcemia, particularly unexplained hypercalcemia, should be accompanied by an intact PTH level as part of the workup. Additional laboratory tests that are helpful include 25-hydroxyvitamin D, creatinine, and possible 24-hour urine calcium levels. Elevated PTH level in the context of hypercalcemia is the classic presentation of PHPT, although serum calcium or PTH level may be in the normal range in some cases.

With moderate to severe elevation of calcium and PTH levels, the diagnosis of PHPT is often straightforward. However, with relatively mild hypercalcemia and PTH elevations, it is important to rule out familial hypocalciuric hypercalcemia (FHH). FHH is an autosomal dominant condition that leads to loss of function of the calcium sensor receptor.[11] There is often a family history of hypercalcemia without evidence of nephrolithiasis or other end-organ damage. FHH is a benign condition that does not require surgery or other interventions. Although there are genetic tests that can be diagnostic, this condition is typically determined by 24-hour urine calcium studies showing levels less than 100 mg in 24 hours as well as a calcium/creatinine ratio less than 0.001.[11]

There are 2 variants of PHPT that should be recognized (**Table 1**). These variants include normocalcemic hyperparathyroidism and normohormonal PHPT. In the case of normocalcemic PHPT, the serum total and ionized calcium levels are within normal limits. Comparatively, if the total level is normal, but the ionized calcium level is elevated, then it is still the classic form of PHPT. The normocalcemic variant of PHPT occurs in approximately 15% of cases.[12] When normocalcemic PHPT is suspected, it is critical to rule out secondary causes of hyperparathyroidism such as chronic renal disease, vitamin D deficiency, and malabsorptive conditions, which cause a physiologic increase in PTH levels.

The normohormonal variant is found when the serum calcium levels are elevated, but the PTH levels are within the normal range. In cases of elevated serum calcium levels, PTH should normally be suppressed and is therefore inappropriately elevated; this is found in 5% to 22% of cases **Table 1**.[12–15]

Patients with PHPT present in 2 different ways: symptomatic or asymptomatic. Symptomatic patients present with conditions such as nephrolithiasis, osteoporosis, and pancreatitis, among others.[16] These conditions are signs of end-organ damage or risk to end organs. Other common symptoms that can affect quality of life include muscle cramps, bone pain, abdominal cramping, fatigue, and melancholy. Surgical resection is the definitive therapy for symptomatic disease. All patients who are symptomatic and are appropriate surgical candidates should be offered surgical resection.

Asymptomatic patients require a more nuanced approach to management. This presentation has been the most common one in the United States for the past several

Table 1 Variants of Primary hyperparathyroidism		
Type of PHPT	Calcium Level	PTH Level
Classic	Elevated	Elevated
Normocalcemic	Normal	Elevated
Normohormonal	Elevated	Normal

decades.[17] However, it must be recognized that even asymptomatic individuals are at risk for complications of the disease. A prospective study demonstrated that at 10 years after diagnosis, 25% of medically managed patients demonstrated disease progression. At 15 years after diagnosis, 37% of medically managed patients demonstrated disease progression.[18] In those who prefer observation or are not ideal surgical candidates, it is reasonable to follow with close observation and serial laboratory evaluation.

LOCALIZATION STUDIES

Several localization studies can be used to identify parathyroid adenomas, including ultrasonography, nuclear medicine studies, computed tomographic (CT) scan, MRI, and a combination approach.

Ultrasonography

The most common imaging modality is ultrasonography. Ultrasonography has a relatively high likelihood of identifying parathyroid adenomas and has the added benefit of being less invasive than other studies and with minimal risk to the patient. This modality can also identify thyroid lesions that may need to be addressed concurrently with the parathyroid lesion. The incidence of concordant thyroid and parathyroid lesions has been reported as 18% in patients who underwent surgery for PHPT.[19] Ultrasonography performed by a skilled operator can be exceptionally accurate, with sensitivity reported as high as 89%, a positive predictive value of 98%, and accurate localization to a specific quadrant of 87%.[20] Most clinicians consider ultrasonography as the initial study of choice for all these reasons (**Fig. 1**)

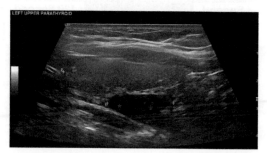

Fig. 1. Ultrasonography of parathyroid adenoma: note the hypoechoic lesion typical of a parathyroid adenoma (red asterik). (*Image courtesy of* Dev Abraham at the University of Utah.)

SESTAMIBI

Sestamibi scintigraphy, also known as a parathyroid scan, historically has had a high positive predictive value and is a first-line study for some clinicians. However, when this technetium scan is used alone, it provides limited anatomic detail and, thus, should be performed with a CT overlay. The sestamibi scan capitalizes on the preferential uptake of sestamibi in hyperactive parathyroid glands, and lack of uptake in normal glands. The positive predictive value can be negatively impacted by concomitant thyroid lesions, which also can have increased uptake of the radiotracer.[21] The overall sensitivity and specificity of sestamibi scan has been reported as 84% and 87%, respectively.[22]

4DCT

Another imaging modality that has gained traction is the use of 4 dimensional computed tomography(4D-CT) (**Fig. 2**), which uses the variable enhancement characteristics of parathyroid adenomas, thyroid tissue, and lymph nodes to differentiate hyperactive parathyroid glands from other structures. Parathyroid adenomas enhance early after iodine-based contrast that washes out quickly, whereas lymph nodes enhance late. Thyroid tissue enhances early but maintains with enhancement. When

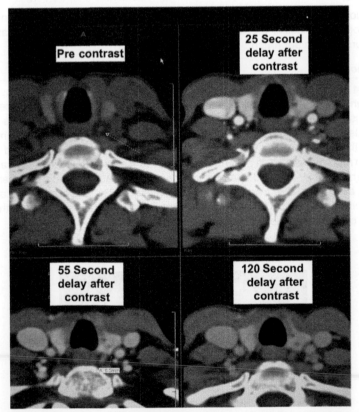

Fig. 2. 4D-CT of parathyroid adenoma: note the changes in contrast enhancement of the left superior parathyroid adenoma (*arrow*). The gland enhances vividly at 25 seconds and then starts to washout at 55 and 120 seconds.

compared with sestamibi scans and ultrasonography, 4D-CT has shown promising improvements in sensitivity, lateralization, and accurate localization to a specific quadrant, with one study reporting a sensitivity of 88%.[23] 4D-CT has been shown to be particularly useful in patients with mild hypercalcemia or small adenomas, reaching statistical significance over sestamibi scan in overall accuracy (73 vs 62%) and hemisphere (66 vs 48%) and quadrant localization (45 vs 29%) in those with serum calcium levels less than 10.8.[24]

MRI

MRI is an additional imaging modality that can be used, typically in combination with others or when others have failed to localize a lesion. In a prospective review of patients who underwent ultrasonography, sestamibi, and MRI, MRI had a sensitivity of 97.8% and specificity of 97.5%, both of which were superior to ultrasonography or sestamibi scan alone. In addition, when combined with ultrasonography, MRI and ultrasonography together identified all enlarged glands in patients with multiglandular disease.[25]

New Techniques in Localization

In more recent years, there has been an attempt to capitalize on the advantages of both the sestamibi nuclear medicine scan and the 4D-CT; this required contrast-enhanced scanning to be coupled with the nuclear medicine imaging. This transition was a fairly simple one, because sestamibi already is performed with a noncontrast CT in most locations. The results have been promising with expected high rates of localization.[26]

PET/CT has also emerged as a new imaging modality. This modality is 18F-fluorocholine PET/CT, and when compared with single-photon emission computed tomography/CT, one study found increasing accuracy of identifying smaller parathyroid adenomas. In addition, PET/CT demonstrated a trend for an increased standard uptake value (SUV) max in patients with parathyroid adenomas versus parathyroid hyperplasia, although this did not reach statistical significance.[27]

Best practice

Ultrasonography followed by 4D-CT versus sestamibi with 4D-CT.[28]

SURGICAL APPROACHES

The first parathyroidectomy was performed by Felix Mandl[29] of Vienna in 1925. From that time, bilateral neck exploration (BNE) was the standard surgical approach and is still an important technique in parathyroid surgery. At present, there have been 2 primary approaches to surgical management of PHPT: 4-gland exploration and localization-directed minimally invasive parathyroidectomy.

Four-Gland Exploration

Four-gland exploration has been a tried and true surgical technique for PHPT. This technique involves an incision on the anterior aspect of the neck with identification of all 4 parathyroid glands. Once all 4 glands have been identified, the decision must be made as to how many glands need to be removed. Historically, surgeons performed the procedure through a sizable incision, but explorations are now routinely performed through incisions that are 3 to 5 cm in length. The advantage of this technique is that it identifies all 4 glands, thereby minimizing the risk that a subclinical parathyroid adenoma or hyperplastic gland is left behind. This technique is often more efficient than minimally invasive parathyroidectomy with intraoperative technique because there is no delay in waiting for intraoperative PTH (iPTH) levels.

There are some disadvantages of this technique. Regardless of how small the incision is, it is still considered a maximally invasive procedure for parathyroid surgery in that it requires bilateral exploration and identification of all 4 glands. Also, it can be challenging if one of the glands is located in an ectopic location. Anatomic studies have found the incidence of ectopic glands to be greater than 40%, whereas surgical experience has shown the incidence to be closer to 15%.[30–32] Although glands can be found anywhere along the course of parathyroid gland embryologic migration, it is important for the parathyroid surgeon to know the most common locations to explore. The incidence of ectopic glands is higher for the inferior glands, which is related to the thymus descending. These glands can be found along the thyrothymic ligament and into the chest within the thymus. Although the superior glands are more reliable, they can be found deep within the tracheoesophageal groove, including into the upper mediastinum or retroesophageal. Also, ectopic glands within the thyroid and along the carotid sheath can occur for both inferior and superior glands (**Fig. 3**). Of note, when inferior glands are not found in the standard location, the surgeon should first follow the thyrothymic ligament and evaluate the superior portion of the thymus in the neck and superior mediastinum (**Fig. 4**). However, glands located more inferiorly in the chest would be impossible to locate with a cervical exploration (**Fig. 5**).

This technique relies on a few important points. First, localization is still important; this is primarily to ensure that any ectopic glands are in locations amenable to cervical exploration. The success rate of traditional 4-gland exploration has repeatedly been shown to be greater than 95%.[8,33] In more recent years, this technique has been

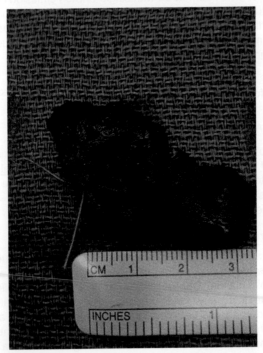

Fig. 3. Intrathyroidal adenoma: the adenoma can be seen adjacent to the cut thyroid tissue.

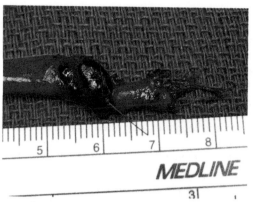

Fig. 4. Thymic adenoma: the adenoma can be seen in the resected thymus and thyrothymic ligament.

coupled with radioguidance. This technique was developed by Martinez and colleagues[34] with the first surgical series reported in 1997 by Norman and Chheda.[35] This technique involves a technetium 99 scan to be performed before undergoing surgery. This scan can serve as a preoperative localization study as well as provide intraoperative guidance. There are 2 techniques that can be used including use of intraoperative radioactivity to detect the quadrant of the adenoma and using the ex vivo activity relative to the background to detect parathyroid adenoma versus normal gland versus other tissue.[36–38]

Intraoperative radioactivity along with the preoperative imaging assists in localizing the parathyroid gland to the correct quadrant or superior mediastinum. Although helpful to identify the general location, this technique may not eliminate the need for other intraoperative confirmations of success, such as evaluation of remaining glands or iPTH.[36]

Over time, radioguided surgery has been popularized for its use in predicting adenomatous tissue versus hyperplasia versus other tissue.[39,40] This approach has been used in lieu of intraoperative frozen section and iPTH monitoring. For this technique, all 4 glands are identified and sampled. Quantitative radioactivity levels are measured with a handheld probe and compared with the background. Parathyroid adenomas are expected to have more than 20% radioactivity as compared with the background. Normal glands, comparatively, will have less than 20% activity. Through this

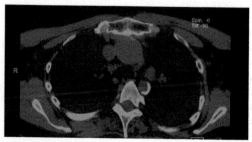

Fig. 5. Thoracic ectopic imaging: the contrasted CT shows an enhancing parathyroid adenoma in the superior mediastinum.

technique, there is an intraoperative detection of parathyroid adenoma. This technique has been described in depth in several studies.[39–42] Data on this technique have shown success rates greater than or equal to 97%.[40,43]

In summary, 4-gland exploration is advantageous in that it identifies all 4 glands and thereby is less likely to miss small subclinical adenomas. This technique also has a higher likelihood of identifying parathyroid hyperplasia. Although parathyroid hyperplasia would not be identified based on the radioguidance, it would be detected on gross visual inspection. This technique has also been reported to improve efficacy, while decreasing costs and length of stay when compared with parathyroidectomy without neck exploration.[44]

The disadvantage of this technique is largely related to the increased invasiveness and potential for increased surgical risk, given the need for identification of all 4 glands and therefore violating surgical planes in close proximity to both recurrent laryngeal nerves. Although not all surgeons agree with the benefits of the radioguided technique, it is a commonly used technique.

Localization-Directed/Minimally Invasive Parathyroidectomy

Focused parathyroidectomy with intraoperative PTH monitoring allows directed removal of a parathyroid adenoma with intraoperative determination that all hyperfunctioning glands have been removed. This technique was initially incorporated in surgery in the early 1990s at the University of Miami.[45,46] This technique takes advantage of the short half-life of PTH (3–5 minutes) and has replaced BNE at most centers across the world. A prerequisite for use of this technique, however, is preexcision localization to direct the side and, ideally, the quadrant of surgery, and this is typically performed with one of the standard preoperative techniques noted earlier.

With an appropriate localization study, the patient will undergo surgery through a small incision with direct approach to the suspicious gland. Intraoperatively, the patient undergoes arterial or venous blood samples for serum PTH levels on a rapid essay. PTH testing occurs before excision and at defined intervals of of 5 to 20 minutes postexcision. A successful surgery, as initially defined by the Miami criterion, will identify a 50% drop from the preexcision PTH at 10 minutes postexcision. Using this technique, cure rates are found to be 97% to 99%.[47–49] Compared with traditional BNE, surgery with iPTH shows an equal to slightly improved success. However, the ability to perform minimally invasive surgery in an ambulatory setting and the associated decrease in operative times, length of stay, morbidity, and costs are significant advantages.[6,47,48,50,51] Over the years, there have been attempts to modify the Miami criterion in an attempt to limit missed multigland disease, improve success rates, and decrease costs. These stricter criteria have included a larger drop of PTH at 10 minutes (>65%–70%), requiring the drop to be within the normal limits of the assay, as well as others.[52–54] Although more restrictive criterion may detect more multigland disease, it will also lead to more BNEs requiring the surgeon to determine hyperfunctioning glands based on visual inspection and the size of the gland. The challenge is that the size of the gland and even the histology do not always predict function.[49,55] Thus, more restrictive criterion may lead to increased explorations and removal of normal functioning glands in the attempt to identify multigland disease.

With the advent of techniques that allow improved localization, better assessment of gland function intraoperatively, and improved detection of surgical cure before ending surgery, the need for traditional BNE has been significantly limited. Use of iPTH monitoring or gamma-probe-directed surgery is a widely practiced and accepted method of performing parathyroidectomy. **Table 2** shows some of the advantages and disadvantages of each technique.

Table 2 Surgical approaches overview		
Surgical Approach	**Pros**	**Cons**
Four-gland exploration	• Identify all glands with or without radioguidance • Lower risk of missing subclinical disease	• More invasive • Bilateral exploration • Risk to bilateral recurrent laryngeal nerves • Still need preoperative imaging to rule out ectopic gland
Minimally invasive	• If localization accurate, can do very targeted dissection	• Need to wait on intraoperative confirmation (PTH levels, pathology) • May still need to do bilateral exploration

Regardless of the technique, one of the factors is the experience of the surgeon. Although many parathyroidectomies may be straightforward, there are intraoperative techniques and challenges in decision making that may lean on the experience of the surgeon in head and neck endocrine surgery.[56–61] It is generally accepted that high-volume thyroid/parathyroid surgeons have improved surgical outcomes; however, high volume is poorly defined. For parathyroid surgery, there are a few studies that specifically look at outcomes related to parathyroid surgical volumes.[56–58,62] Based on the limited data, it appears that increased volume is associated with improved outcomes, lower rates of complications, and decreased costs due to higher likelihood of ambulatory surgery. So, although no strict definition of "low-volume" parathyroid surgeon can be concluded, most studies would suggest less than 15 to 20 parathyroid surgeries per year being low volume and greater than 40 parathyroid surgeries per year being high volume.

Intraoperative Nerve Monitoring

Intraoperative nerve monitoring is a technique that was developed with the intention of decreasing recurrent laryngeal nerve injury. It is more commonly used during thyroid-ectomy than parathyroidectomy alone, and its utility remains a subject of debate. Multiple studies have demonstrated no significant decrease in recurrent laryngeal nerve injury for thyroidectomy and parathyroidectomy, although data for parathyroidectomy alone are lacking.[63]

In addition, the use of intraoperative nerve monitoring for thyroid surgery significantly increases cost, with studies reporting an increase of 5% to 7% total hospital and surgical costs.[63,64] There is no current study looking at exact cost implications during parathyroidectomy alone. Because of these reasons, intraoperative nerve monitoring is not routinely indicated for parathyroid surgery but can be a useful adjunct particularly in revision surgery.

Intraoperative Venous Sampling

For nonlocalizing cases and inability to identify lesions intraoperatively, venous sampling can be helpful. Intraoperative venous sampling allows the ability to lateralize the location of an adenoma based on the difference of PTH levels drawn from bilateral internal jugular veins.[65,66] This technique relies on a greater than 5% difference in PTH level between the 2 samples. One study demonstrated overall sensitivity of bilateral jugular vein PTH sampling of 80%; it additionally localized 57.8% of adenomas that

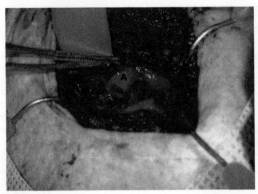

Fig. 6. ICG localization: with administration of indocyanine green, the hypervascular parathyroid adenoma seen noted as a fluorescent lesion, A

had negative preoperative imaging with sestamibi, and aided in identifying lesions when iPTH levels obtained peripherally did not decrease as predicted after removal of glands. In cases in which there is no identification of a suspected adenoma on preoperative imaging, other techniques are sometimes used including sampling of the internal jugular vein preoperatively to guide the side of exploration.

Intraoperative Fluorescence

The highly vascular parathyroid adenomas make them an ideal candidate for use of intraoperative indocyanine green (ICG) immunofluorescence (**Fig. 6**). Hyperactive parathyroid glands tend to take up more ICG than surrounding tissue, which allows for visualization during surgery.[67] This visualization can be limited by bleeding during surgery, which causes ICG to be dispersed throughout the operative field. However, the technology is a promising adjunct to traditional intraoperative methods.[67] Newer techniques are emerging that are taking advantage of the ability of parathyroid glands to autofluoresce. Although intriguing, the use of autofluorescence is not yet defined for parathyroid surgery.

Thoracic

Ectopic parathyroid adenomas can be located in the mediastinum in 22% of ectopic inferior glands and 14% of ectopic superior glands.[32] When these cannot be resected through a traditional cervical incision, it historically required an open approach through a thoracotomy. However, new advances in video-assisted thoracoscopic surgery and robotic thoracic surgery have been increasingly successful for these lesions (**Fig. 7**).

Nonsurgical Approaches

For patients who prefer not to have surgery or are at extremely high surgical risk, there are medical and ablative alternatives. However, surgical resection remains the standard of care. Medical options largely include aggressive hydration, antiresorption medication to protect skeletal integrity, and agents that lower serum calcium levels.[68] Ablative techniques include ethanol, laser, radiofrequency, high-intensity ultrasound, and microwave ablation (MWA). A recent study of 67 patients who underwent MWA showed promising results; however, long-term cure rate remains inferior to surgical resection.[69]

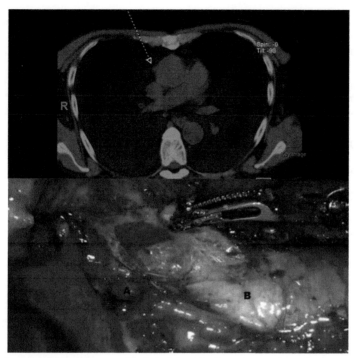

Fig. 7. Robotic thoracic adenoma. (*Top*) A right side thoracic parathyroid adenoma (*arrow*) adjacent to ascending aorta. (*Bottom*) Intraoperative robotic resection; A, parathyroid adenoma; B, ascending aorta. (*Images courtesy of* John Stringham, MD of Department of Surgery, University of Utah Health.)

SUMMARY

Symptomatic PHPT remains a condition cured only by surgical resection. Asymptomatic PHPT can be closely monitored, but upfront surgical resection is reasonable. When working up PHPT, it is critical to rule out familial hypocalciuric hypercalcemia. It is also important to distinguish between the variants of PHPT and rule out secondary or tertiary hyperparathyroidism. Once a diagnosis is secured, preoperative imaging aids in successful minimally invasive parathyroidectomy. Ultrasonography followed by 4D-CT versus sestamibi with 4D-CT is reasonable in most cases. There are alternatives to surgical resection; however, long-term outcomes are inferior. When able, minimally invasive parathyroidectomy is generally preferred. In cases in which an adenoma is unable to be localized either preoperatively or intraoperatively, 4-gland exploration remains the standard of care.

CLINICS CARE POINTS

- PHPT can be classic, normocalcemic, or normohormonal
- Other pathologies causing hypercalcemia or elevated PTH levels must be ruled out
- Appropriate preoperative imaging will aid in minimally invasive parathyroidectomy

- Four-gland exploration remains an important technique, especially if there is an inadequate drop in PTH levels, to resection of presumed adenoma
- Thoracic parathyroid adenomas require a multidisciplinary approach and appropriate surgical planning
- Medical and ablative techniques are alternatives to surgical resection, but remain inferior in efficacy and cure rate

DISCLOSURE

Nothing to disclose.

REFERENCES

1. Yeh MW, Ituarte PH, Zhou HC, et al. Incidence and prevalence of primary hyperparathyroidism in a racially mixed population. J Clin Endocrinol Metab 2013;98: 1122–9.
2. Fisher SB, Perrier ND. Primary hyperparathyroidism and hypertension. Gland Surg 2020;9(1):142–9.
3. Lind L, Ljunghall S. Pre-operative evaluation of risk factors for complications in patients with primary hyperparathyroidism. Eur J Clin Invest 1995;25:955–8.
4. Kalla A, Krishnamoorthy P, Gopalakrishnan A, et al. Primary hyperparathyroidism predicts hypertension: results from the National Inpatient Sample. Int J Cardiol 2017;227:335–7.
5. Trombetti A, Christ ER, Henzen C, et al. Clinical presentation and management of patients with primary hyperparathyroidism of the swiss primary hyperparathyroidism cohort: a focus on neuro-behavioral and cognitive symptoms. J Endocrinol Invest 2016;39(5):567–76.
6. Udelsman R. Six hundred fifty-six consecutive explorations for primary hyperparathyroidism. Ann Surg 2002;235(5):665–72.
7. Walgenbach S, Hommel G, Junginger T. Outcome after surgery for primary hyperparathyroidism: ten-year prospective follow-up study. World J Surg 2000;24:564–70.
8. Allendorf J, DiGorgi M, Spanknebel K, et al. 1112 Consecutive Bilateral Neck Explorations for Primary Hyperparathyroidism. World J Surg 2007;31:2075–80.
9. Barczynski M, Bränström G Dionigi, Mihai R. Sporadic multiple parathyroid gland disease—a consensus report of the European Society of Endocrine Surgeons (ESES). Langenbeck's Arch Surg 2015;400:887–905.
10. Low RA, Katz AD. Parathyroidectomy via bilateral cervical exploration: a retrospective review of 866 cases. Head Neck 1998;20(7):583–7.
11. Lee Janet Y, Shoback Dolores M. Familial hypocalciuric hypercalcemia and related disorders. Best Pract Res Clin Endocrinol Metab 2018;32(Issue 5): 609–19. https://doi.org/10.1016/j.beem.2018.05.004.
12. Kiriakopoulos A, Petralias A, Linos D. Classic primary hyperparathyroidism versus normocalcemic and normohormonal variants: do they really differ? World J Surg 2018;42:992–7.
13. Applewhite Megan K, White Michael G, Tseng Jennifer, et al. Normohormonal primary hyperparathyroidism is a distinct form of primary hyperparathyroidism. Surgery 2017;161(Issue 1):62–9.
14. Mischis-Troussard C, Goudet P, Verges B, et al. Primary hyperparathyroidism with normal serum intact parathyroid hormone levels. QJM: An Int J Med 2000;93(6): 365–7.

15. Wallace Lucy B, Parikh Rikesh T, Ross Louis V, et al. The phenotype of primary hyperparathyroidism with normal parathyroid hormone levels: How low can parathyroid hormone go? Surgery 2011;150(6):1102–12.

16. Khan AA, Hanley DA, Rizzoli R, et al. Primary hyperparathyroidism: review and recommendations on evaluation, diagnosis, and management. A Canadian and international consensus. Osteoporos Int 2017;1–19.

17. Silverberg SJ, Clarke BL, Peacock M, et al. Current issues in the presentation of asymptomatic primary hyperparathyroidism: proceedings of the Fourth International Workshop. J Clin Endocrinol Metab 2014;99(10):3580–94. Summarizes data on the various traditional and nontraditional manifestations of PHPT according to the expert panel consensus of the Fourth International Workshop on the Management of Asymptomatic Primary Hyperparathyroidism. This report provides information on the natural history of PHPT, geographic differences of predominant phenotypes and various organ system involvement of PHPT.

18. Rubin MR, Bilezikian JP, McMahon DJ, et al. The natural history of primary hyperparathyroidism with or without parathyroid surgery after 15 years. J Clin Endocrinol Metab 2008;93(9):3462–70.

19. Bentrem DJ, Angelos P, Talamonti MS, et al. Is preoperative investigation of the thyroid justified in patients undergoing parathyroidectomy for hyperparathyroidism? Thyroid 2002;12(12):1109–12.

20. Gilat H, Cohen M, Feinmesser R, et al. Minimally invasive procedure for resection of a parathyroid adenoma: the role of preoperative high-resolution ultrasonography. J Clin Ultrasound 2005;33(6):283–7.

21. Wojtczak B, Syrycka J, Kaliszewski K, et al. Surgical implications of recent modalities for parathyroid imaging. Gland Surg 2020;9(Suppl 2):S86–94.

22. Nafisi Moghadam R, Amlelshahbaz AP, Namiranian N, et al. Comparative diagnostic performance of ultrasonography and 99mTc-sestamibi scintigraphy for parathyroid adenoma in primary hyperparathyroidism; systematic review and meta- analysis. Asian Pac J Cancer Prev 2017;18(12):3195–200.

23. Rodgers SE, Hunter GJ, Hamberg LM, et al. Improved preoperative planning for directed parathyroidectomy with 4-dimensional computed tomography. Surgery 2006;140(6):932–40 [discussion: 940-1].

24. Eichhorn-Wharry LI, Carlin AM, Talpos GB. Mild hypercalcemia: an indication to select 4-dimensional computed tomography scan for preoperative localization of parathyroid adenomas. Am J Surg 2011;201(3):334–8 [discussion: 338].

25. Argirò R, Diacinti D, Sacconi B, et al. Diagnostic accuracy of 3T magnetic resonance imaging in the preoperative localisation of parathyroid adenomas: comparison with ultrasound and 99mTc-sestamibi scans. Eur Radiol 2018;28(11):4900–8.

26. Neumann DR, Obuchowski NA, Difilippo FP. Preoperative 123I/99mTc-sestamibi subtraction SPECT and SPECT/CT in primary hyperparathyroidism. J Nucl Med 2008;49(12):2012–7.

27. Beheshti M, Hehenwarter L, Paymani Z, et al. ^{18}F-Fluorocholine PET/CT in the assessment of primary hyperparathyroidism compared with ^{99m}Tc-MIBI or ^{99m}Tc-tetrofosmin SPECT/CT: a prospective dual-centre study in 100 patients. Eur J Nucl Med Mol Imaging 2018;45(10):1762–71.

28. Solorzano CC, Carneiro-Pla D. Minimizing cost and maximizing success in the preoperative localization strategy for primary hyperparathyroidism. Surg Clin North Am 2014;94(3):587–605.

29. Mandl F. Klinisches und experimentelles zur frage der lokalisierten und generalisierten ostitis fibrosa: unter besonderer berücksichtigung der therapie der letzteren. Teil 2. Arch Klin Chir 1926;143:245–8.

30. Wang CA. The anatomic basis of parathyroid surgery. Ann Surg 1976;183:271–5.
31. Mendoza V, Ramirez C, Espinoza AE, et al. Characteristics of ectopic parathyroid glands in 145 cases of primary hyperparathyroidism. Endocr Pract 2010;16: 977–81.
32. Phitayakorn R, McHenry CR. Incidence and location of ectopic abnormal parathyroid glands. Am J Surg 2006;191(3):418–23.
33. van Heerden JA, Grant CS. Surgical treatment of primary hyperparathyroidism: an institutional perspective. World J Surg 1991;15(6):688–92.
34. Martinez DA, King DR, Romshe C, et al. Intraoperative identification of parathyroid gland pathology: a new approach. J Pediatr Surg 1995;30:1306–9.
35. Norman J, Chheda H. Minimally invasive parathyroidectomy facilitated by intraoperative Nucl mapping. Surgery 1997;122:998–1003.
36. Westerdahl J, Bergenfelz A. Sestamibi scan-directed parathyroid surgery: potentially high failure rate without measurement of intraoperative parathyroid hormone. World J Surg 2004;28(11):1132–8.
37. Westra WH, Pritchett DD, Udelsman R, et al. Intraoperative confirmation of parathyroid tissue during parathyroid exploration. Am J Surg Pathol 1998;22(5): 538–44.
38. Satchie B, Chen H. Radioguided techniques for parathyroid surgery. Asian J Surg 2005;28(2):77–81.
39. Murphy C, Norman J. The 20% rule: A simple, instantaneous radioactivity measurement defines cure and allows elimination of frozen sections and hormone assays during parathyroidectomy. Am Assoc Endocr Surgeons 1999;126(6). https://doi.org/10.1067/msy.2099.101578.
40. McGreal G, Winter DC, Sookhai S, et al. Minimally invasive, radioguided surgery for primary hyperparathyroidism. Ann Surg Oncol 2001;8(10):856–60.
41. Angelos P. An initial experience with radioguided parathyroid surgery. Am J Surg 2000;180:475–8.
42. Takami H, Takayama J, Ikeda Y, et al. Section 1. Parathyroid: minimally invasive radioguided parathyroidectomy 2002;56(1):37–40.
43. Livingston CD. Radioguided parathyroidectomy is successful in 98.7% of selected patients. Endocr Pract 2014;20(4):305–9.
44. Goldstein RE, Blevins L, Delbeke D, et al. Effect of minimally invasive radioguided parathyroidectomy on efficacy, length of stay, and costs in the management of primary hyperparathyroidism. Ann Surg 2000;231(5):732–42.
45. Irvin GL 3rd, Dembrow VD, Prudhomme DL. Operative monitoring of parathyroid gland hyperfunction. Am J Surg 1991;162:299–302.
46. Irvin GL 3rd, Prudhomme DL, Deriso GT, et al. A new approach to parathyroidectomy. Ann Surg 1994;219:574–9.
47. Westerdahl J, Lindblom P, Bergenfelz A. Measurement of Intraoperative Parathyroid Hormone Predicts Long-term Operative Success. Arch Surg 2002;137(2): 186–90.
48. Grant CS, Thompson G, Farley D, et al. Primary Hyperparathyroidism surgical management since the introduction of minimally invasive parathyroidectomy: mayo clinic experience. Arch Surg 2005;140(5):472–9.
49. Irvin GL 3rd, Carneiro DM, Solorzano CC. Progress in the operative management of sporadic primary hyperparathyroidism over 34 years. Ann Surg 2004;239(5): 704–11.
50. Chen Herbert, Sokoll Lori J, Udelsman Robert. Outpatient minimally invasive parathyroidectomy: A combination of sestamibi-SPECT localization, cervical

block anesthesia, and intraoperative parathyroid hormone assay. Surgery 1999; 126(6):1016–22.

51. Fahy BN, Bold RJ, Beckett L, et al. Modern parathyroid surgery: a cost-benefit analysis of localizing strategies. Arch Surg 2002;137:917–22.

52. Chiu B, Sturgeon C, Angelos P. Which intraoperative parathyroid hormone assay criterion best predict operative success? A study of 352 consecutive patients. Arch Surg 2006;141:483–7.

53. Barczynski M. Minimally invasive parathyroidectomy without intraoperative parathyroid hormone monitoring: When and why? J Postgrad Med 2009;55:239–40.

54. Clerici T, Brandle M, Lange J, et al. Impact on intraoperative parathyroid hormone monitoring on the prediction of multiglandular parathyroid disease. World J Surg 2004;28:187–92.

55. McGill J, Sturgeon C, Kaplan SP, et al. How does the operative strategy for primary hyperparathyroidism impact the findings and cure rate? A comparison of 800 parathyroidectomies. J Am Coll Surg 2008;207:246–9.

56. Stavrakis AI, Ituarte PH, Ko CY, et al. Surgeon volume as a predictor of outcomes in inpatient and outpatient endocrine surgery. Surgery 2007;142(6):887–99 [discussion 887-99].

57. Neychev VK, Ghanem M, Blackwood SL, et al. Parathyroid surgery can be safely performed in a community hospital by experienced parathyroid surgeons: A retrospective cohort study. Int J Surg 2016;27:72–6.

58. Sosa JA, Bowman HM, Tielsch JM, et al. The importance of surgeon experience for clinical and economic outcomes from thyroidectomy. Ann Surg 1998;228(3): 320–30.

59. Meltzer C, Klau M, Gurushanthaiah D, et al. Surgeon Volume in parathyroid surgery—surgical efficiency, outcomes, and utilization. JAMA Otolaryngol Head Neck Surg 2017;143(8):843–7.

60. Adam MA, Roman SA, Sosa JA. Outpatient parathyroidectomy. In: Stack B Jr, Bodenner D, editors. Medical and surgical treatment of parathyroid diseases. Cham (Switzerland): Springer; 2017.

61. Tuggle Charles T, Roman Sanziana A, Wang Tracy S, et al. Pediatric endocrine surgery: Who is operating on our children? Surgery 2008;144(6):869–77.

62. Erinjeri N, Udelsman R. Volume-outcome relationship in parathyroid surgery. Best Pract Res Clin Endocrinol Metab 2019;33(5):101287.

63. Ghani U, Assad S, Assad S. Role of intraoperative nerve monitoring during parathyroidectomy to prevent recurrent laryngeal nerve injury. Cureus 2016;8(11): e880.

64. Dionigi G, Bacuzzi A, Boni L, et al. Visualization versus neuromonitoring of recurrent laryngeal nerves during thyroidectomy: what about the costs? World J Surg 2012;36(4):748–54.

65. Taylor J, Fraser W, Banaszkiewiz P, et al. Lateralization of parathyroid adenomas by intra-operative parathormone estimation. J R Coll Surg Edinb 1996;41:174–7.

66. Ito F, Sippel R, Lederman J, et al. The utility of intra-operative bilateral venous sampling with rapid parathyroid hormone testing. Ann Surg 2007;245:959–63.

67. Spartalis E, Ntokos G, Georgiou K, et al. Intraoperative indocyanine green (ICG) angiography for the identification of the parathyroid glands: current evidence and future perspectives. Vivo 2020;34(1):23–32.

68. Cetani F, Saponaro F, Marcocci C. Non-surgical management of primary hyperparathyroidism. Best Pract Res Clin Endocrinol Metab 2018;32(6):821–35.

69. Wei Y, Peng L, Li Y, et al. Clinical Study on safety and efficacy of microwave ablation for primary hyperparathyroidism. Korean J Radiol 2020;21(5):572–81.

Update on Tracheostomy and Upper Airway Considerations in the Head and Neck Cancer Patient

Grace M. Wandell, MD, MS*, Albert L. Merati, MD,
Tanya K. Meyer, MD

KEYWORDS

- Head and neck cancer • Airway management • Tracheostomy • Difficult airway
- Tracheotomy

KEY POINTS

- Elective and emergent management of the difficult airway in HNC patient requires multidisciplinary collaboration between the surgeon and anesthesiologist.
- There are several choices of endotracheal tubes and methods for oxygenation during laryngeal surgery, such as intubation, intermittent apnea, THRIVE, and jet ventilation.
- More research is needed to define the risk factors and appropriate indications for peritreatment tracheotomy in head and neck cancer.
- There is increasing evidence that early tracheotomy reduces the rate of ventilator-associated pneumonia and results in system-wide cost improvements and quality measures.
- More high-quality studies are needed to investigate optimal tracheostomy care. Multidisciplinary teams and institutional protocls may improve tracheostomy outcomes.

INTRODUCTION

As a considerable amount of morbidity in the head and neck cancer (HNC) population arises because of airway compromise, the surgeon caring for these patients should anticipate the possibility of managing a difficult airway.[1,2] Patients with head, neck, and tracheal pathology account for 39% of major perioperative airway events.[1,3,4] Aside from perioperative airway concerns, tracheostomy is frequently performed in this population.[5] Although HNC is far from the most common indication, tracheostomy is one of the most common surgical procedures,[6] with over 100,000 tracheotomies

Department of Otolaryngology—Head & Neck Surgery, University of Washington, 1959 Northeast Pacific, Suite BB1165, PO Box 356515, Seattle, WA 98195-6515, USA
* Corresponding author.
E-mail address: gracemwandell@gmail.com

Surg Clin N Am 102 (2022) 267–283
https://doi.org/10.1016/j.suc.2021.12.005
0039-6109/22/© 2021 Elsevier Inc. All rights reserved.

Abbreviations	
HNC	Head and neck cancer
VL	Videolaryngoscopy
FOI	Fiberoptic intubation
CI	Confidence Interval
OR	Odds ratio
OT	Open tracheotomy
PDT	Percutaneous dilational tracheotomy
BMI	Body mass index
AT	Awake tracheotomy
CMS	Center for Medicare & Medicaid Service
RCT	Randomized controlled trial
TRPI	Tracheostomy-related pressure injuries
ACV	Above cuff vocalization
ET	Early tracheotomy
LT	Late tracheotomy

being performed in the United States each year.[7] The main indications for tracheotomy include respiratory failure with ventilator dependence, airway obstruction, and pulmonary toilet.[7,8] Given these considerations, this article seeks to update the surgeon caring for HNC patients on recent advancements and literature in the management of the difficult airway and adult tracheostomy.

DIFFICULT AIRWAY MANAGEMENT
Medical Treatments

The adult airway is approximately 13 to 15 cm long and 11 to 25 mm wide, with the narrowest point at the level of the vocal folds.[9] In the patient with respiratory distress related to upper airway compromise, medications such as heliox, steroids, and racemic epinephrine may bridge patients before intubation or establishment of a surgical airway. Heliox is a biologically inert gas, which decreases work of breathing and improves gas delivery to the lungs by reducing airflow resistance and transforming turbulent airflow into laminar airflow.[10] Although more widely studied in pediatric populations and most benefits being reported in small, observational studies, it is a safe temporizing measure.[10] Also better studied in the setting of pediatric croup, racemic epinephrine used in adult upper airway obstruction appears to be a safe and effective adjunct (0.5 mL of a 2% solution diluted in a volume of 2 to 4 mL, given every 4 hours).[11]

Corticosteroids continue to play an important role in airway management.[12] There have been meta-analyses of randomized controlled trials (RCTs) examining and supporting the use of corticosteroids to prevent reintubation and airway events at the time of extubation.[13–16] Kuriyama and colleagues (2017) performed a meta-analysis of 11 RCTs including 2472 subjects on this topic and concluded that prophylactic corticosteroids reduce the incidence of postextubation airway events and reintubation, particularly among patients at high risk for reintubation as determined using a cuff-leak test.[16] The minimal leak test (MLT) is the most common method for reporting the endotracheal cuff pressure. It involves completely deflating the cuff and then listening for an audible leak.[17] In the high-risk group without a cuff leak, pre-extubation treatment with corticosteroids was associated with relative risks of 0.34 (95% CI 0.24–0.48) and 0.35 (95% CI 0.020–0.64) for reducing postextubation airway events and reintubation, respectively.[16] Given these considerations, pre-extubation steroids may be considered in HNC patients at high risk of extubation failure.

Intubation Considerations

It is important to choose the optimal type and size of endotracheal tube (ETT) for an HNC patient with a difficult airway or a patient undergoing a head and neck procedure.[18] A microlaryngeal tube is frequently used in laryngeal surgery because of its small internal diameter (4–6 mm), yet maintaining a standard adult tube length and cuff volume.[18] A metallic reinforced tube prevents kinking when put under pressure in the case of oral and nasal surgeries. A laser-safe ETT, wrapped with either aluminum or copper foil and containing 2 cuffs in case of inadvertent damage, should be considered in laryngeal surgeries involving the use of laser to prevent balloon damage and airway fire.[18] When choosing an ETT size, height is cited as the main determinant; however, many patients are still inappropriately intubated with larger than necessary tubes, particularly women and individuals with a heigh of less than 160 cm.[19] Surgeons and anesthetists should work closely together when selecting the appropriate tube for a patient undergoing surgery for HNC.

After selection of the appropriate ETT, one must consider the appropriate intubation method in these patients. Videolaryngoscopy (VL) and awake or sedated fiberoptic intubation (FOI) are frequently considered.[20,21] VL provides a wider field of visualization during intubation while being rigid, making it less easily displaced by airway obstruction as compared with FOI.[20] In comparison to traditional direct laryngoscopy, in a Cochrane review of 3100 participants, VL was associated with less laryngeal trauma (OR 0.68, 95% CI 0.48–0.96) and postoperative dysphonia (OR 0.56, 95% CI 0.36–0.88).[22] These benefits have led to widespread adoption of this tool during both difficult and routine intubation.

Although helpful in difficult airway patients, VL alone may be inadequate among some HNC patients. Hyman and colleagues (2020) performed a prospective, observational study defining the grade and quality of the view obtained with VL among 100 patients who were deemed at higher risk of a difficult intubation (due to a history of head and neck mass or prior radiation) and preselected to undergo FOI. . They examined the view obtained using VL and found that in one-third of patients, no view was possible, whereas FOI was successful in 99% of cases.[3] Though observational data, their results indicate that despite its popularity, VL may be limited for a large proportion of patients in the HNC population and FOI should be considered.

Awake FOI should be considered when there are risk factors for a difficult intubation such as trismus, known airway obstruction, dental damage, obesity, history of difficult mask ventilation, or when excessive cervical spine manipulation should be avoided.[23] Providers should avoid deep sedation and muscle relaxant in patients with a fixed airway obstruction.[24] Sedation may be administered during awake intubation, to enhance patient comfort and cooperation, with medications such as fentanyl, midazolam, and remifentanil infusion.[23] In addition, providers can administer local anesthesia in the form of a lidocaine gargle, nebulizer, or a superior laryngeal nerve block.[23]

Alternatives to Intubation—the Tubeless Surgical Field

Aside from traditional endotracheal intubation, there are several alternatives for oxygenation and ventilation which providers may consider during head and neck surgery, particularly laryngeal surgery. Although traditionally used in the pediatric population, general anesthesia with spontaneous ventilation can be used during laryngeal suspension for glottic, subglottic, and tracheal procedures.[25] Transnasal Humidified Rapid Insufflation Ventilatory Exchange (THRIVE) is another option when the airway is shared between the anesthetist and surgeon.[20,26] It delivers warm, humidified high-flow oxygen during apneic oxygenation and uses aventilatory mass flow, a phenomenon where the gradients between oxygen and carbon dioxide at the alveoli generate a negative pressure gradient.[27,28] Both techniques avoid obscuring the posterior glottis and trauma associated with intermittent intubation during apneic laryngeal surgery,[26] and can maintain oxygenation during surgical procedures lasting less than 1 hour.[28] Downsides of using a tubeless technique include hypercapnia, lack of a definitive airway, and the risk of aspiration.[28] THRIVE should be avoided in patients with significant nasal pathology or skull base fractures, and both techniques are more challenging in obese patients.[28]

Jet ventilation is another attractive alternative when the surgical field resides in the airway.[29] Jet ventilation provides a short burst of oxygen at a high pressure via a small catheter,[18,30] and can be performed at the level of the supraglottis, glottis, or trachea.[18] Transtracheal jet ventilation may be used in an emergent, airway cases where intubation is not possible.[18] In jet ventilation, there is no standardized system for expiration.[29] Therefore, the risks of jet ventilation include inadequate ventilation leading to hypercapnia, laryngospasm, misdirection of the jet leading to barotrauma, and dangerously increasing the intrathoracic pressure, which could result in increases in intracranial pressure and cardiovascular compromise, due to a lack of ability for the patient to exhale due to a narrowed glottis.[18,29,31] In a recently published study examining 371 patients receiving supraglottic jet ventilation during endoscopic treatment of laryngotracheal stenosis, intraoperative complications occurred in less than 1% of patients and acute postoperative complications occurred in 3% of patients.[32] Although many avoid using jet ventilation among patients with a higher body mass index, most studies do not demonstrate an increased risk of complications.[32]

TRACHEOSTOMY AND SURGICAL AIRWAYS
Preoperative Planning in HNC Patients

Whether for long-term or short-term airway management or pulmonary hygiene, tracheotomy is frequently performed in the HNC population, although appropriate indications for tracheotomy in this population continue to be debated. In laryngeal cancer specifically, radiation therapy may result in chronic aspiration, laryngeal edema, and chondronecrosis which may require tracheotomy placement before, during, or after radiation therapy.[33] Advanced T stage and vocal cord paralysis before radiation treatment increase the risk of the need for tracheotomy after chemoradiation in laryngeal cancer.[34] In a small observational cohort, Du and colleagues (2016)[35] advocate that tumor debulking may be an alternative to tracheotomy in T3/T4 supraglottic tumors.

For other HNCs, tracheotomy was once the standard for most complex, microvascular reconstructions of the upper aerodigestive tract.[36,37] However, the data on the benefits and indications for tracheotomy in this population are mixed, and many are now advocating for the discontinuation of routine tracheotomy, as the downsides of tracheotomy may outweigh the benefits, such a prolonged hospitalization and time to oral intake.[38] Based on the available evidence, elective tracheostomy placement may be considered in patients with a bulky free flap reconstruction, a history of radiotherapy, and a history of smoking.[5] A small, retrospective analysis of the benefits of tracheotomy in patients undergoing microsurgical tissue transfer for oropharyngeal cancer found that the procedure was associated with fewer ventilated days ($P = .005$).[39] However, in an American College of Surgeons National Surgical Quality Improvement Program (NSQIP) multivariate analysis of 861 patients, a lack of tracheotomy was not associated with 30-day airway-specific complications.[36] The diverse nature of these patients' procedures, cancers, and risk-factors for airway difficulties postoperatively makes this question particularly challenging and deserves future study.

Tracheotomy Procedural Variations and Approaches

When the surgeon decides tracheotomy is appropriate, there are 2 main methods of performing tracheotomy: open tracheotomy (OT) or percutaneous dilation tracheotomy (PDT). With either approach, the procedure creates an opening, ideally between the second and third tracheal rings, from the neck to the airway.[40]

Open tracheotomy

The detailed steps of OT are available in other literature and are only briefly described here.[41] OT is performed by creating a 2 to 3 cm horizontal incision approximately 1 cm below the cricoid. Next, the superficial layer of the deep cervical fascia is divided, avoiding the anterior jugular venous vasculature. The strap muscles and thyroid isthmus are divided. A cricoid hook should be placed to secure the airway into the operative field. After the surgeon bluntly removes the pretracheal fascia, they must communicate with their anesthesiologist before entering the airway. If the patient is anesthetized and intubated, the ETT is temporarily deflated before creating a horizontal incision between the second and third tracheal rings. Once the airway is visualized, the anesthesiologist partially retracts the ETT and the surgeon inserts the new tracheostomy tube and confirms end-tidal CO_2 return. The main benefits of OT include improved anatomic exposure and hemostasis.[42]

Various techniques can be used when making the tracheal incision. When OT is performed during neck dissection in the HNC patient, some advocate for using a vertical midline incision to avoid contaminating the neck dissection wound.[43] A Bjork flap is an inferiorly based inverted U-shaped tracheal flap placed through the second, third, and fourth rings, which is affixed to the skin or deep cervical fascia.[43–45] It theoretically reduces trach tube shear forces on tracheal mucosa and makes tracheostomy changes safer and easier in a maturing stoma.[46] Others advocate for its use because of less risk of tracheal stenosis.[43] Within institutions, practices of performing the Bjork flap vary widely.[47] In a retrospective, single-institution study comparing 217 patients receiving a Bjork flap versus a tracheal window, Bjork flaps were more frequently performed in patients with larger tracheostomy tubes (size 8 vs 6), who needed tracheostomy for long-term ventilation, had a history of stroke, and had a higher BMI. There were no differences in rates of postoperative bleeding or successful decannulation.[46] Overall, the literature on the benefits and downsides of the Bjork flap is sparse.

Percutaneous dilatational tracheotomy

Although OT has been the standard for years, PDT, with continued adaptations and modernization, is gaining popularity and becoming widely accepted.[6,47,48] The basic steps include placing a 2 cm incision from the inferior border of the cricoid toward the sternal notch, blunt dissection through the subcutaneous tissue, passing a seeking needle between the first and second or second and third tracheal rings, and confirming needle placement via bronchoscopic visualization or aspiration of air. Then, using the Seldinger technique, a guidewire is passed into the airway, the tract is dilated, and the tracheostomy tube is passed into the airway and secured.[41] Variations of the procedure include making the tracheotomy using a landmark-guided technique, bronchoscopy guidance, or ultrasound guidance. Using bronchoscopy during PDT minimizes the risk of posterior tracheal wall injury. However, one downside of bronchoscopy-guided PDT is the risk of disturbing ventilation.[49] In a meta-analysis of 4 RCTs, ultrasound-guided PDT demonstrated comparable rates of major complications compared with other techniques, although less complications compared with anatomic landmark-guided PDT.[50]

There is variability in provider attitudes about contraindications to percutaneous tracheostomy. Some cite obesity and large thyroid goiters as relative contraindications[47,51] Many studies have evaluated the safety and complications of PDT as compared with OT. PDT has been reported to have more frequent postoperative bleeding (6.6% vs 1.9%). However, Halum and colleagues (2012) compared bleeding rates between different tracheotomy techniques with and without stay sutures in a multi-institutional retrospective analysis of complications and found that stay sutures were less frequently used in PDT, and that using them during both OT and PDT was associated with lower bleeding rates.[8] Therefore, it is plausible that the less frequent use of stay sutures could contribute to the higher bleeding rates observed with PDT, although this would need to be confirmed with an RCT. In 2016, a Cochrane review of 16 RCTs and 4 quasi-RCTs found no difference between the 2 approaches in terms of overall mortality, major bleeding, accidental decannulation, or a difficult tube exchange.[51] However, PDT was associated with lower rates of infection, delayed wound healing, tracheal stenosis, fistulas, and scarring.[51] Despite these findings, a large analysis of 8682 patients in the New York database found PDT to be associated with slightly higher mortality (OR 1.18, CI 1.03–1.33, $P = .12$) when adjusting for comorbidity using the Charleston Comorbidity Index and other confounding factors.[48]

PDTs are frequently performed by nonotolaryngologists and their rise has been associated with decreasing numbers of tracheotomies being performed by otolaryngologists.[6,52] In recent years, the numbers of tracheotomies performed by otolaryngology residents has declined as well, which may be correlated with the rise in popularity of the PDT.[53] As otolaryngologists are responsible for managing the complications of all forms of tracheotomy and that there is some evidence that PDT may be more cost-effective,[42] otolaryngologists and surgeons should become comfortable with both techniques.

Awake tracheostomy

An awake tracheostomy (AT) refers to performing a tracheostomy under local anesthesia with minimal sedation to allow a patient with a compromised airway to continue to manage their airway reflexes.[54] A current head and neck malignancy, especially with increased risk of bleeding during intubation, is the most common indication for performing an AT. Other indications for AT include subglottic stenosis, angioedema, and neck infection or hematoma.[54] In a retrospective review of 1469 patient charts, AT was associated with increased 6.2 higher odds of pneumothorax and/or pneumomediastinum.[55]

RISKS AND COMPLICATIONS

Complications in tracheotomy are cited to occur 4.3% to 40% of cases,[40] with the most agreed upon rate being approximately 15%.[56] Tracheotomy complications are typically divided into immediate, early, and late categories.[55,56] The immediate complications of subcutaneous emphysema and pneumothorax occur in 0-9% and 0-4% of cases, respectively, and may be avoided by minimizing pretracheal dissection and adhering to the midline airway.[56] The most common early postoperative complication is bleeding (2%–4% of cases), followed by mucus plugging (2.7%) and unplanned decannulation (0.35%–15%).[40,56] Using a tube with an inner cannula may safeguard against mucus plugging.[56] Patients with chronic neurologic disorders, chronic tracheostomy, and cervical lordosis are at increased risk of the feared complication of tracheoinnominate fistula,[57] which may be treated with sternotomy or endovascular approaches.[58]

Both intubation and tracheostomy cause long-term airway complications, such as posterior glottic stenosis and subglottic/tracheal stenosis from intubation and stenosis at the level of the trach site in tracheostomy. Airway stenosis is the most common late complication and reports of its incidence vary widely in the literature from 1% to 20%.[8,59] A national study of an emergency department database identified that 1.05% of patients who had previously undergone tracheostomy re-presented to the hospital with symptoms of tracheal stenosis.[60] Tracheal stenosis from tracheostomy tube forms due to granulation tissue formation around the stoma and tube and cartilage damage, and is frequently associated with tracheomalacia.[61] A recent retrospective review of 91 patients undergoing surgical tracheostomy with preprocedure and postprocedure CT imaging available reported the rate of tracheal stenosis to be 8.8%. The only risk factor they identified for developing stenosis was a history of prior tracheostomy.[59] A larger review at one center of 1656 patients found that greater than 10 days of orotracheal intubation, ETT cuff pressure greater than 30, and obesity were risk factors for tracheal stenosis.[62] Tracheostomy tube cuff pressure above 30 mm Hg leads to ischemia of the tracheal mucosa, resulting in ulceration and cartilage damage.[63] Other long-term complications that greatly impact patient quality of life and experience include those related to prolonged cuff inflation, such as laryngeal desensitization, secretion stasis, uncoordinated glottic closure, decreased cough strength, and overall increased aspiration risk.[64]

EMERGENT SURGICAL AIRWAY

In the acute setting, when the previously described methods have failed to secure an airway in the HNC patient, and bag masking is not possible, an emergent surgical airway must be established. Options include a cricothyroidotomy or a slash tracheotomy.[23] The cricothyroid membrane is a 6-8 mm vertically tall fibroelastic tissue which spans the space between the cricoid and thyroid cartilage.[23] Cricothyrotomy involves palpating the cricothyroid membrane, creating a 1 to 3 cm midline vertical incision in the overlying skin, creating and dilating a 1 cm horizontal incision through the cricothyroid membrane, and rapidly inserting an endotracheal tube. Once the patient is stabilized, and if it is anticipated that the patient will require prolonged intubation, the cricothyrotomy must be converted to a formal tracheostomy.[23] Alternatively, emergent tracheostomy or a "slash trach" may be performed.[65] Upper airway obstruction due to malignancy is the most common indication for emergent AT.[66] Emergent tracheotomies are more frequently performed by otolaryngologists or surgeons, whereas a range of health care professionals (EMTs, nurses, anesthesiologists) perform cricothyroidotomy in emergency situations.[65,67]

Many advocate for the use of a cricothyrotomy procedure because it may be simpler, faster, and less prone to complications compared with an emergent tracheotomy.[23] The complication rate of all types of emergent surgical airways is as high as 28%, with reported risks of this procedure including subcutaneous emphysema, pneumothorax, pneumonia, tracheoesophageal fistula, and granulation tissue formation.[68] In multivariate analysis of 402 cases of emergent tracheotomies performed by otolaryngologists, a history of neck pathology and the tracheotomy being performed outside the operating room were risk factors for increased complication rates.[68] In addition, laryngeal cancer is a significant risk factor for unplanned tracheotomy during panendoscopy.[69] Two systematic reviews compared complications rates between the procedures and found that they were mostly similar.[65,70] However, emergent cricothyrotomy was associated with 0.21 lower odds (95% CI 0.2–0.2) of late complications compared with emergent tracheotomy.[65]

Tracheostomy Management and Postoperative Care

There is significant variation among institutions, surgeons, and proceduralists performing tracheostomy regarding appropriate postoperative management.[63] As tracheostomy is one of the most common procedures and is performed by a variety of physicians, there is growing recognition of the need to improve the safety and quality of this procedure across hospital systems using multidisciplinary teams, bundles, pathways, and collaborative approaches.[71–76] The Global Tracheostomy Collaborative (GTC) is one important international collaboration, data-sharing, and quality improvement effort to improve tracheostomy care and outcomes.[71,76] The GTC includes 45 member hospitals that develop educational events and materials, share data, and compare outcomes.[76] Recent guidelines support the use of tracheostomy care bundles which include a specialized order set, decannulation protocol, and tracheostomy rounds.[77] Multidisciplinary tracheostomy teams including a physician, speech-language pathologist, and respiratory therapist have been also shown to reduce tracheostomy adverse events and time to decannulation, and increase the use of speaking valves.[77] For example, Masood and colleagues (2018) implemented a standardized postoperative tracheostomy care protocol at one academic medical center among 247 patients, delineating a standardized protocol and training on proper suctioning and cleaning. Postprotocol rapid response rates decreased by 8.7% (95% CI 0.2%–18%) and decreased mucus plugging by 6.0% (95% CI 1.3%–12.2%).[78]

Sutures

At the time of surgery, many surgeons frequently place temporary outer phalange sutures to secure the tracheostomy tube to the skin during the immediate postoperative period.[8] This practice has been associated with reduced rates of postoperative bleeding in a retrospective study of complications.[8] Lee and colleagues (2014) advocate for the use of stay sutures in a small study of 104 individuals due to one accidental decannulation that was fatal in a patient who did not have stay sutures.[79] However, accidental decannulation rates have been cited to be similar between patients with and without stay sutures in other studies.[8,80,81] Fine and colleagues (2020) published a retrospective cohort of 1355 patients undergoing tracheotomy and found that within 7 postoperative days, there were no significant differences in the incidence of dislodgement or accidental decannulation for patients with nonsutured ties (1.5%) and sutured ties (1.1%).[80] The benefit of stay sutures requires study in a prospective or randomized study.

Tracheostomy tube change and care

Patterns in the appropriate timing of tracheostomy tube change also vary widely.[82] One of the main theoretic reasons for a tube change is to reduce the rate of potential infection associated with a foreign body. Yet, Kumarasinghe and colleagues (2020) demonstrated that there are no differences in bacterial colonization in patients undergoing changes greater or less than every 4 weeks.[83] One observational historical cohort study at one institution, demonstrated that changing tracheostomy tubes every 2 weeks was associated with a reduction in the number of patients requiring surgical intervention to address granulation tissue.[63] A randomized cross-over study measuring bacterial colonization indicates that tracheostomy inner cannulas may be cleaned with either chlorhexidine or detergent-based products with similar efficacy.[84] The appropriate timing and frequency of tracheostomy tube change requires further study.

Cuff deflation

Deflation of the tracheostomy cuff is important to facilitate communication, normal airflow, begin the path toward decannulation, and limit tracheal wall injury. Excessive secretions in patients with a tracheostomy, often due to underlying dysphagia and an inability to swallow secretions, may limit cuff deflation trials.[64] A subglottic drainage port may be used to assess the volume of pooled secretions and may reduce the incidence of ventilator-associated pneumonia (VAP). Alternatively, sublingual atropine drops (1% 1–2 drops TID), glycopyrrolate (5 ug/kg IV or SC TID), hyoscine (1.5 mg patch q72 hours), and salivary botox may be used to control oropharyngeal secretions.[64]

Wound infection and pressure injury

Preventing infectious and visible complications related to tracheostomy placement is important for patients and hospital systems. Although preoperative antibiotics are frequently administered, an RCT of 159 patients found that they have no impact on the rate of stomal wound infection.[85] Preventing wound breakdown associated with tracheostomy is key: the Centers for Medicare and Medicaid Services (CMS) designate pressure ulcers as key events for hospital reimbursement and tracheostomy-related pressure injuries (TRPI) occur in approximately 10% of patients.[86] Moist dressings, including foam, hydrocolloid, Mepilex Ag, and hydrogel dressings, are sometimes used to prevent tracheostomy device-related pressure wounds.[87] However, the literature differs about the efficacy of these dressings. An RCT of 80 patients compared regular gauze to foam dressings. There were 7.5% less infections in the foam group, although this difference was not statistically significant.[88] However, in a meta-analysis of 10 studies comparing moist dressings to sterile gauze, moist dressings decreased the risk of infection by 59% and pressure ulcer formation by 78%.[87] There is mounting evidence that institutional initiatives to decrease TRPI may be helpful.[86,89] A multidisciplinary tracheostomy pressure injury prevention team implemented a quality improvement initiative which reduced rates of TRPI. Their protocol included placement of stay sutures with air knots, a soft foam Velcro collar, and a Duo-Derm hydrocolloid dressing underneath the superior phalange at the time of the procedure. They removed stay sutures on postoperative day 3 and changed hydrophilic foam dressings once every 3 days.[86]

Voice

Patients with a tracheostomy tube may have difficulty vocalizing. For patients without the need for mechanical ventilation or frequent suctioning, one-way speaking valves, often referred to as Passy Muir valves (PMVs), can be attached to the outer cuffless tracheostomy tube to allow exhalational airflow via the vocal cords and a speaking voice.[90] Fenestrated tracheostomy tubes are sometimes used to allow for phonation and promote successful decannulation, and may be considered as a method of phonation in patients expected to need long-term ventilation.[90] However, they are infrequently used because of significant downsides, including greater rates of granulation formation and subcutaneous emphysema if malpositioned.[90] Alternatively, above cuff vocalization (ACV), also known as a "talking tracheostomy," may be used in patients in whom the cuff cannot be deflated.[64,91] ACV involves applying air via a subglottic port in a tracheostomy tube and may have positive effects on communication, swallowing, coughing, and quality of life among patients with tracheostomy.[91]

Decannulation

There is geographic variance in ultimate decannulation rates, but the estimated rate in the United States is 8%.[8,71] There have been few RCTs on the optimal protocol for decannulation.[92] In a nonblinded controlled trial of 330 patients, Hernández and colleagues (2020) demonstrated that the frequency of suctioning in a 24-hour period versus a 24-hour capping trial may better predict decannulation and lead to earlier decannulation times.[93] A small RCT demonstrated that suture closure of the tracheostomy after decannulation may improve swallowing outcomes.[94]

Dysphagia

Dysphagia with a tracheostomy is common, occurring in many as 80% of individuals.[95] Although many advocate for the avoidance of oral intake while the tracheostomy cuff is inflated, systematic reviews and meta-analyses analyzing the topic cite varying results, insufficient evidence, and bias in the existing studies that make examining the impact of cuff inflation on swallowing physiology untenable.[95,96] The modified Evan's blue dye test (MEBDT), which involves mixing blue dye with water or food, is commonly used to evaluate aspiration risk in patient with tracheostomies. However, methodologic inconsistencies between the few existing studies evaluating the sensitivity and specificity of this test require further study to delineate its value.[97]

Tracheostomy Outcomes

Early versus late tracheotomy

There is significant debate and interest over the benefits to the patient and hospital system of early tracheotomy (ET) versus late tracheotomy (LT). ET is frequently defined as <7 to 10 days since intubation, but ranges from 3 to 10 days.[8,98] One of the most frequently debated benefits of ET is whether it decreases the rate of VAP.[99] A review of 124,990 Nationwide insurance claims of tracheostomy established a linear correlation between increasing time to tracheostomy and VAP and found that ET (ET defined as <10 days) was associated with a small reduction in VAP (OR 0.92, 95% CI 0.87–0.98).[100] In a recently published meta-analysis, Chorath and colleagues (2021) found that among greater than 3000 patients, ET (<7 days from intubation) was associated with a lower incidence of VAP (OR 0.59, 95% CI 0.35–0.99).[99]

ET has been associated with hospital system improvements in several studies such as shorter ICU and hospital stays.[99,101] Chorath and colleagues also found that ET was associated with fewer ICU days (mean difference −6.25 days, 95% CI −11.22 to −1.28).[99] In multivariate analysis in the Nationwide Insurance claims study adjusting for demographics, comorbidities, insurance, and patient income, ET significantly reduced length of stay (effect ratio: 0.77, 95% CI 0.76–0.79) and hospital costs (effect ratio: 0.78, 95% CI 0.77–0.79).[100] A cost analysis modeling study estimated that ET reduces hospital costs by $4316 (95% CI: 403–8229), mostly due to reductions in ICU length of stay.[102]

Disparities

Increasing awareness is mounting surrounding disparities in the type and quality of tracheostomy care received among minority populations. Hispanic patients with tracheostomy have been shown to have a higher 30-day mortality rate, despite having a lower rate of comorbidity compared with other ethnic groups.[103] Black, Hispanic, and Medicaid-insured patients have longer hospital stays when tracheotomy is performed and may be less likely to receive ET.[48] Given these associations and mounting evidence that ET improves outcomes, providers will need to pay attention to and investigate the factors driving these disparities among vulnerable populations.

SUMMARY

Patients with HNC represent some of the most challenging difficult airway cases; however, there are several technologies that are improving management of these patients. Choosing the best airway plan during surgery for the patient with HNC involves close communication between the surgeon and anesthesiologist. Although tracheostomy is one of the oldest and most commonly performed procedures, there are increasing and needed efforts focused on tracheostomy process improvements which will be useful for providers caring for patients with HNC. There is mounting evidence that ET is associated with improvements in VAP, hospital stay, and cost savings. Future research should focus on methodologically improved studies examining the impact of variations in post-tracheostomy care. There is increasing recognition of the need for the development of collaborative and multidisciplinary tracheostomy bundles to improve safety and quality of this common procedure.[71] These improvements will hopefully lead to improved outcomes among HNC patients undergoing tracheotomy.

DISCLOSURE

The authors have nothing to disclose.

REFERENCES

1. Artime CA, Roy S, Hagberg CA. The difficult airway. Otolaryngol Clin North Am 2019;52(6):1115–25. https://doi.org/10.1016/j.otc.2019.08.009.
2. Mohamedbhai H, Ali S, Dimasi I, et al. TRACHY score: a simple and effective guide to management of the airway in head and neck cancer. Br J Oral Maxillofac Surg 2018;56(8):709–14. https://doi.org/10.1016/j.bjoms.2018.07.015.
3. Hyman JB, Apatov D, Katz D, et al. A prospective observational study of video laryngoscopy use in difficult airway management. Laryngoscope 2020;131(1): 82–6. https://doi.org/10.1002/lary.28637.
4. Cook TM, Woodall N, Frerk C. Major complications of airway management in the UK: results of the Fourth National Audit Project of the Royal College of Anaesthetists and the Difficult Airway Society. Part 1: anaesthesia. Br J Anaesth 2011; 106(5):617–31. https://doi.org/10.1093/bja/aer058.
5. Yi CT, Zhang W, Yu Y, et al. Scoring system for selective tracheostomy in head and neck surgery with free flap reconstruction. Head Neck 2020;42(3):476–84. https://doi.org/10.1002/hed.26028.
6. Patel HH, Siltumens A, Bess L, et al. The decline of tracheotomy among otolaryngologists: a 14-year review. Otolaryngol Neck Surg 2015;152(3):465–9. https://doi.org/10.1177/0194599814563513.
7. Reed CR, Haines KL, Agarwal SK. Tracheostomy. In: Current surgical therapy. Elsevier, Inc; 2020. p. 1394–404. https://doi.org/10.1016/B978-0-323-64059-6. 00253-X.
8. Halum SL, Ting JY, Plowman EK, et al. A multi-institutional analysis of tracheotomy complications. Laryngoscope 2012;122(1):38–45. https://doi.org/10.1002/lary.22364.
9. Gaissert HA, Burns J. The compromised airway: tumors, strictures, and tracheomalacia. Surg Clin North Am 2010;90(5):1065–89. https://doi.org/10.1016/j.suc.2010.06.004.
10. McGarvey JM, Pollack CV. Heliox in airway management. Emerg Med Clin North Am 2008;26(4):905–20. https://doi.org/10.1016/j.emc.2008.07.007.
11. Macdonnel S, Timmins A, Watson JD. Adrenaline administered via a nebulizer in adult patients with upper airway obstruction. Anaesthesia 1995;50(1):35–6. https://doi.org/10.1111/j.1365-2044.1995.tb04510.x.
12. Cavallone LF, Vannucci A. Extubation of the difficult airway and extubation failure. Anesth Analg 2013;116(2):368–83. https://doi.org/10.1213/ANE. 0b013e31827ab572.

13. François B, Bellissant E, Gissot V, et al. 12-H pretreatment with methylprednisolone versus placebo for prevention of postextubation laryngeal oedema: a randomised double-blind trial. Lancet 2007;369(9567):1083–9. https://doi.org/10.1016/S0140-6736(07)60526-1.

14. Fan T, Wang G, Mao B, et al. Prophylactic administration of parenteral steroids for preventing airway complications after extubation in adults: meta-analysis of randomised placebo controlled trials. BMJ 2008;337(7678):1088–91. https://doi.org/10.1136/bmj.a1841.

15. Jaber S, Jung B, Chanques G, et al. Effects of steroids on reintubation and postextubation stridor in adults: meta-analysis of randomised controlled trials. Crit Care 2009;13(2):1–11. https://doi.org/10.1186/cc7772.

16. Kuriyama A, Umakoshi N, Sun R. Prophylactic corticosteroids for prevention of postextubation stridor and reintubation in adults: a systematic review and meta-analysis. Chest 2017;151(5):1002–10. https://doi.org/10.1016/j.chest.2017.02.017.

17. Selman Y, Arciniegas R, Sabra JM, et al. Accuracy of the minimal leak test for endotracheal cuff pressure monitoring. Laryngoscope 2020;130(7):1646–50. https://doi.org/10.1002/lary.28328.

18. Cherian VT, Vaida SJ. Airway management in laryngeal surgery. Oper Tech Otolaryngol Head Neck Surg 2019;30(4):249–54. https://doi.org/10.1016/j.otot.2019.09.005.

19. Cao AC, Rereddy S, Mirza N. Current practices in endotracheal tube size selection for adults. Laryngoscope 2020;131(9):1967–71. https://doi.org/10.1002/lary.29192.

20. Moore A, Schricker T. Awake videolaryngoscopy versus fiberoptic bronchoscopy. Curr Opin Anaesthesiol 2019;32(6):764–8. https://doi.org/10.1097/ACO.0000000000000771.

21. Mark L, Herzer K, Akst S, et al. General considerations of anesthesia and management of the difficult airway. 7th edition. Elsevier Inc; 2010. https://doi.org/10.1016/b978-0-323-05283-2.00010-0.

22. Lewis SR, Butler AR, Parker J, et al. Videolaryngoscopy versus direct laryngoscopy for adult patients requiring tracheal intubation: a cochrane systematic review. Br J Anaesth 2017;119(3):369–83. https://doi.org/10.1093/bja/aex228.

23. Karle WE, Schindler JS. Surgical management of the difficult adult airway. 7th edition. Elsevier Inc; 2010. https://doi.org/10.1016/b978-0-323-05283-2.00011-2.

24. Yadav N, Ahmad SA, Kumar N, et al. Airway management of a post tracheostomy stenosis patient with respiratory difficulty make sure you have fibre optic guidance before administering muscle relaxant! Trauma Mon 2016;21(3):e20927. https://doi.org/10.1056/nejm196103232641203.

25. Yoo MJ, Joffe AM, Meyer TK. Tubeless total intravenous anesthesia spontaneous ventilation for adult suspension microlaryngoscopy. Ann Otol Rhinol Laryngol 2018;127(1):39–45. https://doi.org/10.1177/0003489417744223.

26. Benninger MS, Zhang ES, Chen B, et al. Utility of transnasal humidified rapid insufflation ventilatory exchange for microlaryngeal surgery. Laryngoscope 2021;131(3):587–91. https://doi.org/10.1002/lary.28776.

27. Patel A, Nouraei SAR. Transnasal Humidified Rapid-Insufflation Ventilatory Exchange (THRIVE): a physiological method of increasing apnoea time in patients with difficult airways. Anaesthesia 2015;70(3):323–9. https://doi.org/10.1111/anae.12923.

28. Huang L, Dharmawardana N, Badenoch A, et al. A review of the use of trans-nasal humidified rapid insufflation ventilatory exchange for patients undergoing surgery in the shared airway setting. J Anesth 2020;34(1):134–43. https://doi.org/10.1007/s00540-019-02697-3.

29. Galmén K, Harbut P, Freedman J, et al. The use of high-frequency ventilation during general anaesthesia: an update. F1000Res 2017;6. https://doi.org/10.12688/f1000research.10823.1.

30. Chhetri DK, Long JL. Airway management and CO2 laser treatment of subglottic and tracheal stenosis using flexible bronchoscope and laryngeal mask anesthesia. Oper Tech Otolaryngol Head Neck Surg 2011;22(2):131–4. https://doi.org/10.1016/j.otot.2011.01.001.

31. Jaquet Y, Monnier P, Van Melle G, et al. Complications of different ventilation strategies in endoscopic laryngeal surgery: a 10-year review. Anesthesiology 2006;104(1):52–9. https://doi.org/10.1097/00000542-200601000-00010.

32. Rodney JP, Shinn JR, Amin SN, et al. Multi-institutional analysis of outcomes in supraglottic jet ventilation with a team-based approach. Laryngoscope 2021; 131(10):2292–7. https://doi.org/10.1002/lary.29431.

33. Armstrong WB, Vokes DE, Tjoa T, et al. Malignant tumors of the larynx. In: Cummings otolaryngology: head and neck surgery. 7th edition. Elsevier Inc; 2021. p. 1564–95.e11. https://doi.org/10.1016/B978-0-323-61179-4.00105-8.

34. Lavo JP, Ludlow D, Morgan M, et al. Predicting feeding tube and tracheotomy dependence in laryngeal cancer patients. Acta Otolaryngol 2017;137(3): 326–30. https://doi.org/10.1080/00016489.2016.1245864.

35. Du E, Smith RV, Ow TJ, et al. Tumor debulking in the management of laryngeal cancer airway obstruction. Otolaryngol Head Neck Surg 2016;155(5):805–7. https://doi.org/10.1177/0194599816661326.

36. Cramer JD, Samant S, Greenbaum E, et al. Association of airway complications with free tissue transfer to the upper aerodigestive tract with or without tracheotomy. JAMA Otolaryngol Head Neck Surg 2016;142(12):1177–83. https://doi.org/10.1001/jamaoto.2016.2002.

37. Dawson R, Phung D, Every J, et al. Tracheostomy in free-flap reconstruction of the oral cavity: can it be avoided? A cohort study of 187 patients. ANZ J Surg 2021;91(6):1246–50. https://doi.org/10.1111/ans.16762.

38. Coyle MJ, Tyrrell R, Godden A, et al. Replacing tracheostomy with overnight intubation to manage the airway in head and neck oncology patients: towards an improved recovery. Br J Oral Maxillofac Surg 2013;51(6):493–6. https://doi.org/10.1016/j.bjoms.2013.01.005.

39. Meier J, Wunschel M, Angermann A, et al. Influence of early elective tracheostomy on the incidence of postoperative complications in patients undergoing head and neck surgery. BMC Anesthesiol 2019;19(1):1–6. https://doi.org/10.1186/s12871-019-0715-9.

40. Bontempo LJ, Manning SL. Tracheostomy emergencies. Emerg Med Clin North Am 2019;37(1):109–19. https://doi.org/10.1016/j.emc.2018.09.010.

41. Kraft SM, Schindler JS. Tracheotomy. In: Cummings otolaryngology - head and neck surgery. 7th edition Philadelphia, PA; 2021. doi:10.1016/B978-0-323-61179-4.00007-7

42. Levin R, Trivikram L. Cost/benefit analysis of open tracheotomy, in the OR and at the bedside, with percutaneous tracheotomy. Laryngoscope 2001;111(7): 1169–73. https://doi.org/10.1097/00005537-200107000-00008.

43. Malata CM, Foo ITH, Simpson KH, et al. An audit of Bjork flap tracheostomies in head and neck plastic surgery. Br J Oral Maxillofac Surg 1996;34(1):42–6. https://doi.org/10.1016/S0266-4356(96)90134-5.

44. Stathopoulos P, Stassen L. A modification of the Bjork flap in tracheostomies for head and neck cancer patients. J Stomatol Oral Maxillofac Surg 2018;119(5): 444–5. https://doi.org/10.1016/j.jormas.2018.04.018.

45. Au JK, Heineman TE, Schmalbach CE, et al. Should adult surgical tracheos-tomies include a Bjork flap? Laryngoscope 2017;127(3):535–6. https://doi.org/10.1002/lary.26305.

46. Kennedy MM, Abdel-Aty Y, Lott DG. Comparing tracheostomy techniques: Bjork flap vs. tracheal window. Am J Otolaryngol Head Neck Med Surg 2021;42(6): 103030. https://doi.org/10.1016/j.amjoto.2021.103030.

47. Henry LE, Paul EA, Atkins JH, et al. Institutional analysis of intra- and post-operative tracheostomy management for risk reduction. World J Otorhinolar-yngol Head Neck Surg 2021. https://doi.org/10.1016/j.wjorl.2021.02.004.

48. Yang A, Gray ML, McKee S, et al. Percutaneous versus surgical tracheostomy: timing, outcomes, and charges. Laryngoscope 2018;128(12):2844–51. https://doi.org/10.1002/lary.27334.

49. Plata P, Gaszyński T. Ultrasound-guided percutaneous tracheostomy. Anaesthe-siol Intensive Ther 2019;51(2):126–32.

50. Gobatto ALN, Besen BAMP, Cestari M, et al. Ultrasound-guided percutaneous dilational tracheostomy: a systematic review of randomized controlled trials and meta-analysis. J Intensive Care Med 2020;35(5):445–52. https://doi.org/10.1177/0885066618755334.

51. Brass P, Hellmich M, Ladra A, et al. Percutaneous techniques versus surgical techniques for tracheostomy. Cochrane Database Syst Rev 2016;2016(7). https://doi.org/10.1002/14651858.CD008045.pub2.

52. Bowen AJ, Nowacki AS, Benninger MS, et al. Is tracheotomy on the decline in otolaryngology? A single institutional analysis. Am J Otolaryngol Head Neck Med Surg 2018;39(2):97–100. https://doi.org/10.1016/j.amjoto.2017.12.017.

53. Lesko D, Showmaker J, Ukatu C, et al. Declining otolaryngology resident training experience in tracheostomies: case log trends from 2005 to 2015. Oto-laryngol Head Neck Surg 2017;156(6):1067–71. https://doi.org/10.1177/0194599817706327.

54. Sagiv D, Nachalon Y, Mansour J, et al. Awake tracheostomy: indications, com-plications and outcome. World J Surg 2018;42(9):2792–9. https://doi.org/10.1007/s00268-018-4578-x.

55. Bathula SS, Srikantha L, Patrick T, et al. Immediate postoperative complications in adult tracheostomy. Cureus 2020;12(12). https://doi.org/10.7759/cureus.12228.

56. Goldenberg D, Ari EG, Golz A, et al. Tracheotomy complications: a retrospective study of 1130 cases. Otolaryngol Head Neck Surg 2000;123(4):495–500. https://doi.org/10.1067/mhn.2000.105714.

57. Tateyama M, Konno M, Takano R, et al. A computed tomographic assessment of tracheostomy tube placement in patients with chronic neurological disorders: the prevention of tracheoarterial fistula. Intern Med 2019;58(9):1251–6. https://doi.org/10.2169/internalmedicine.1158-18.

58. O'Malley TJ, Jordan AM, Prochno KW, et al. Evaluation of endovascular interven-tion for tracheo-innominate artery fistula: a systematic review. Vasc Endovascu-lar Surg 2021;55(4):317–24. https://doi.org/10.1177/1538574420980625.

59. James P, Parmar S, Hussain K, et al. Tracheal stenosis after tracheostomy. Br J Oral Maxillofac Surg 2021;59(1):82–5. https://doi.org/10.1016/j.bjoms.2020. 08.036.

60. Johnson RF, Saadeh C. Nationwide estimations of tracheal stenosis due to tracheostomies. Laryngoscope 2019;129(7):1623–6. https://doi.org/10.1002/lary. 27650.

61. Zias N, Chroneou A, Tabba MK, et al. Post tracheostomy and post intubation tracheal stenosis: Report of 31 cases and review of the literature. BMC Pulm Med 2008;8:1–9. https://doi.org/10.1186/1471-2466-8-18.

62. Li M, Yiu Y, Merrill T, et al. Risk factors for posttracheostomy tracheal stenosis. Otolaryngol Head Neck Surg 2018;159(4):698–704. https://doi.org/10.1177/ 0194599818794456.

63. Wallace S, McGrath BA. Laryngeal complications after tracheal intubation and tracheostomy. BJA Educ 2021;21(7):250–7. https://doi.org/10.1016/j.bjae. 2021.02.005.

64. Yaremchuk K. Regular tracheostomy tube changes to prevent formation of granulation tissue. Laryngoscope 2003;113(1):1–10. https://doi.org/10.1097/ 00005537-200301000-00001.

65. Zasso FB, You-Ten KE, Ryu M, et al. Complications of cricothyroidotomy versus tracheostomy in emergency surgical airway management: a systematic review. BMC Anesthesiol 2020;20(1):1–10. https://doi.org/10.1186/s12871-020-01135-2.

66. Fang CH, Friedman R, White PE, et al. Emergent awake tracheostomy - the five-year experience at an urban tertiary care center. Laryngoscope 2015;125(11): 2476–9. https://doi.org/10.1002/lary.25348.

67. Lipton G, Stewart M, McDermid R, et al. Multispecialty tracheostomy experience. Ann R Coll Surg Engl 2020;102(5):343–7. https://doi.org/10.1308/ RCSANN.2019.0184.

68. Jotic AD, Milovanovic JP, Trivic AS, et al. Predictors of complications occurrence associated with emergency surgical tracheotomy. Otolaryngol Head Neck Surg 2021;164(2):346–52. https://doi.org/10.1177/0194599820947001.

69. Eissner F, Haymerle G, Brunner M. Risk factors for acute unplanned tracheostomy during panendoscopy in HNSCC patients. PLoS One 2018;13(12):1–8. https://doi.org/10.1371/journal.pone.0207171.

70. DeVore EK, Redmann A, Howell R, et al. Best practices for emergency surgical airway: a systematic review. Laryngoscope Investig Otolaryngol 2019;4(6): 602–8. https://doi.org/10.1002/lio2.314.

71. Brenner MJ, Pandian V, Milliren CE, et al. Global Tracheostomy Collaborative: data-driven improvements in patient safety through multidisciplinary teamwork, standardisation, education, and patient partnership. Br J Anaesth 2020;125(1): e104–18. https://doi.org/10.1016/j.bja.2020.04.054.

72. Cherney RL, Pandian V, Ninan A, et al. The Trach Trail: a systems-based pathway to improve quality of tracheostomy care and interdisciplinary collaboration. Otolaryngol Head Neck Surg 2020;163(2):232–43. https://doi.org/10. 1177/0194599820917427.

73. McGrath BA, Wallace S, Lynch J, et al. Improving tracheostomy care in the United Kingdom: results of a guided quality improvement programme in 20 diverse hospitals. Br J Anaesth 2020;125(1):e119–29. https://doi.org/10.1016/j. bja.2020.04.064.

74. Bonvento B, Wallace S, Lynch J, et al. Role of the multidisciplinary team in the care of the tracheostomy patient. J Multidiscip Healthc 2017;10:391–8. https://doi.org/10.2147/JMDH.S118419.

75. Divo MJ. Post-tracheostomy care: bundle up for success! Respir Care 2017; 62(2):246–7. https://doi.org/10.4187/respcare.05410.

76. Bedwell JR, Pandian V, Roberson DW, et al. Multidisciplinary tracheostomy care: how collaboratives drive quality improvement. Otolaryngol Clin North Am 2019; 52(1):135–47. https://doi.org/10.1016/j.otc.2018.08.006.

77. Mussa CC, Gomaa D, Rowley DD, et al. AARC clinical practice guideline: management of adult patients with tracheostomy in the acute care setting. Respir Care 2021;66(1):156–69. https://doi.org/10.4187/respcare.08206.

78. Masood MM, Farquhar DR, Biancaniello C, et al. Association of standardized tracheostomy care protocol implementation and reinforcement with the prevention of life-threatening respiratory events. JAMA Otolaryngol Head Neck Surg 2018;144(6):527–32. https://doi.org/10.1001/jamaoto.2018.0484.

79. Lee SH, Kim KH, Woo SH. The usefulness of the stay suture technique in tracheostomy. Laryngoscope 2015;125(6):1356–9. https://doi.org/10.1002/lary.25083.

80. Fine KE, Wi MS, Kovalev V, et al. Comparing the tracheostomy dislodgement and complication rate of non-sutured neck tie to skin sutured neck tie fixation. Am J Otolaryngol Head Neck Med Surg 2020;42(1):102791. https://doi.org/10.1016/j.amjoto.2020.102791.

81. Zein Eddine SB, Carver TW, Karam BS, et al. Neither skin sutures nor foam dressing use affect tracheostomy complication rates. J Surg Res 2021;260:116–21. https://doi.org/10.1016/j.jss.2020.11.066.

82. Tabaee A, Lando T, Rickert S, et al. Practice patterns, safety, and rationale for tracheostomy tube changes: a survey of otolaryngology training programs. Laryngoscope 2007;117(4):573–6. https://doi.org/10.1097/MLG.0b013e318030455a.

83. Kumarasinghe D, Wong EH, Duvnjak M, et al. Colonization rates of tracheostomy tubes associated with the frequency of tube changes. ANZ J Surg 2020; 90(11):2310–4. https://doi.org/10.1111/ans.15970.

84. Björling G, Belin AL, Hellström C, et al. Tracheostomy inner cannula care: a randomized crossover study of two decontamination procedures. Am J Infect Control 2007;35(9):600–5. https://doi.org/10.1016/j.ajic.2006.11.006.

85. Sittitrai P, Siriwittayakorn C. Perioperative antibiotic prophylaxis in open tracheostomy: a preliminary randomized controlled trial. Int J Surg 2018;54:170–5. https://doi.org/10.1016/j.ijsu.2018.04.047.

86. Carroll DJ, Leto CJ, Yang ZM, et al. Implementation of an interdisciplinary tracheostomy care protocol to decrease rates of tracheostomy-related pressure ulcers and injuries. Am J Otolaryngol Head Neck Med Surg 2020;41(4):102480. https://doi.org/10.1016/j.amjoto.2020.102480.

87. Yue M, Lei M, Liu Y, et al. The application of moist dressings in wound care for tracheostomy patients: a meta-analysis. J Clin Nurs 2019;28(15–16):2724–31. https://doi.org/10.1111/jocn.14885.

88. Ahmadinegad M, Lashkarizadeh MR, Ghahreman M, et al. Efficacy of dressing with absorbent foam versus dressing with gauze in prevention of tracheostomy site infection. Tanaffos 2014;13(2):13–9.

89. O'Toole TR, Jacobs N, Hondorp B, et al. Prevention of tracheostomy-related hospital-acquired pressure ulcers. Otolaryngol Head Neck Surg (United States) 2017;156(4):642–51. https://doi.org/10.1177/0194599816689584.

90. Pandian BV, Boisen S, Matthews S, et al. Speech and safety in tracheostomy patients receiving mechanical ventilation: a systematic review. Am J Crit Care 2019;28(6):441–50.
91. Mills CS, Michou E, King N, et al. Evidence for above cuff vocalization in patients with a tracheostomy: a systematic review. Laryngoscope 2021. https://doi.org/10.1002/lary.29591.
92. Singh RK, Saran S, Baronia AK. The practice of tracheostomy decannulation-A systematic review. J Intensive Care 2017;5(1). https://doi.org/10.1186/s40560-017-0234-z.
93. Hernández Martínez G, Rodriguez M-L, Vaquero M-C, et al. High-flow oxygen with capping or suctioning for tracheostomy decannulation. N Engl J Med 2020;383(11):1009–17. https://doi.org/10.1056/nejmoa2010834.
94. Brookes JT, Hadi S, Diamond C, et al. Prospective randomized trial comparing the effect of early suturing of tracheostomy sites on postoperative patient swallowing and rehabilitation. J Otolaryngol 2006;35(2):77–82.
95. Skoretz SA, Anger N, Wellman L, et al. A systematic review of tracheostomy modifications and swallowing in adults. Dysphagia 2020;35(6):935–47. https://doi.org/10.1007/s00455-020-10115-0.
96. Goff D, Patterson J. Eating and drinking with an inflated tracheostomy cuff: a systematic review of the aspiration risk. Int J Lang Commun Disord 2019; 54(1):30–40. https://doi.org/10.1111/1460-6984.12430.
97. Béchet S, Hill F, Gilheaney Ó, et al. Diagnostic accuracy of the modified evan's blue dye test in detecting aspiration in patients with tracheostomy: a systematic review of the evidence. Dysphagia 2016;31(6):721–9. https://doi.org/10.1007/s00455-016-9737-3.
98. Koch T, Hecker B, Hecker A, et al. Early tracheostomy decreases ventilation time but has no impact on mortality of intensive care patients: a randomized study. Langenbeck's Arch Surg 2012;397(6):1001–8. https://doi.org/10.1007/s00423-011-0873-9.
99. Chorath K, Hoang A, Rajasekaran K, et al. Association of early vs late tracheostomy placement with pneumonia and ventilator days in critically Ill patients: a meta-analysis. JAMA Otolaryngol Head Neck Surg 2021;78229:1–10. https://doi.org/10.1001/jamaoto.2021.0025.
100. Villwock JA, Jones K. Outcomes of early versus late tracheostomy: 2008-2010. Laryngoscope 2014;124(8):1801–6. https://doi.org/10.1002/lary.24702.
101. Altman KW, Ha TAN, Dorai VK, et al. Tracheotomy timing and outcomes in the critically Ill: complexity and opportunities for progress. Laryngoscope 2021; 131(2):282–7. https://doi.org/10.1002/lary.28657.
102. Herritt B, Chaudhuri D, Thavorn K, et al. Early vs. late tracheostomy in intensive care settings: impact on ICU and hospital costs. J Crit Care 2018;44:285–8. https://doi.org/10.1016/j.jcrc.2017.11.037.
103. Bahethi R, Park C, Yang A, et al. Influence of insurance status and demographic factors on outcomes following tracheostomy. Laryngoscope 2021;131(7): 1463–7. https://doi.org/10.1002/lary.28967.

Workup and Management of Thyroid Nodules

Derek A. Escalante, MD*, Kelly G. Anderson, MD

KEYWORDS

- Thyroid nodule • Ultrasound • Fine needle aspiration biopsy

KEY POINTS

- As the detection of thyroid nodules increases, so does the need for awareness of their management.
- Although they are extremely common, most thyroid nodules are clinically insignificant.
- The initial management of a thyroid nodule includes laboratories to evaluate for hypo or hyperthyroidism and ultrasound.
- Ultrasound features guide the recommendation for fine needle aspiration (FNA). Further management should be based either on FNA results (for those nodules meeting criteria for biopsy) or ultrasound features (for those nodules not meeting criteria for biopsy).
- Clinical goals should be to identify malignancies while avoiding overtreatment and employing a holistic, tailored approach to patients.

INTRODUCTION

An understanding of the management of thyroid nodules is imperative for today's surgeon. Thyroid nodules are extremely common. Even surgeons who do not practice endocrine surgery will likely find themselves managing patients who have had nodules incidentally discovered on cross-sectional imaging for other disease processes (often termed "incidentalomas").[1]

Prevalence

A landmark study in 1955 examined 821 thyroid glands at autopsy and determined that half harbored nodules, despite the absence of clinically evident thyroid disease during the patients' lifetime.[2] More recently, a study performing thyroid ultrasound on 635 patients undergoing routine preventive health checks detected thyroid nodules in 68% of patients.[3]

The increasing accessibility of various imaging modalities in the past 30 years has resulted in more frequent detection of incidental thyroid nodules (**Fig. 1**). Incidental

Madigan Army Medical Center Otolaryngology-Head & Neck Surgery, Tacoma, Washington, USA
* Corresponding author.
E-mail address: derek.a.escalante.mil@mail.mil

Surg Clin N Am 102 (2022) 285–307
https://doi.org/10.1016/j.suc.2021.12.006
0039-6109/22/Published by Elsevier Inc.

surgical.theclinics.com

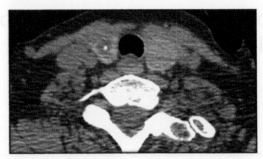

Fig. 1. CT spine of an 83-year-old woman who presented to the emergency room after a ground-level fall, demonstrating an incidental right thyroid nodule (*).

thyroid nodules have been reported in 25% of chest computed tomography (CT) scans, 19.6% of carotid doppler ultrasounds, 16% of neck CTs, and 2% of PET scans in patients without known thyroid disease.[4–7] Though they are exceedingly common, only about 5% of nodules harbor malignancy.[8] Despite increased thyroid nodule detection and the consequent rise in the incidence of thyroid cancer, mortality from thyroid cancer remains low at approximately 0.5 deaths per 100,000 people **(Fig. 2)**.[9] Well-differentiated thyroid cancer (WDTC), which includes both papillary and follicular cancer, constitutes the vast majority of thyroid cancers.

Goals of Management: a less Is More Approach

The widespread detection and subsequent workup of incidental thyroid nodules have raised concerns regarding overdiagnosis and overtreatment of nodules and low-risk thyroid cancers that would be inconsequential to the health or mortality of a patient if gone undetected.[10] The evaluation and management of thyroid nodules and differentiated thyroid carcinoma have therefore evolved to embrace a more conservative approach as it has become evident that the rise in the incidence of differentiated thyroid carcinoma is attributed to the increased detection of small tumors without a preponderance for harm.[11] Management of thyroid nodules has pivoted toward a higher threshold for surgery, less extensive surgery, and the consideration of active surveillance for low-risk disease.

The US Preventive Services Task Force now advises against routine thyroid cancer screening in asymptomatic adults to minimize harmful treatment effects that outweigh potential benefits.[12] The de-escalation of diagnostic and treatment intensity is also apparent in the most recent iteration of the American Thyroid Association (ATA) Guidelines, which advocates for less surveillance, consideration of less extensive surgeries, and less radioactive iodine (RAI) than its previous publications.[13] The ATA guidelines acknowledge minimization of overtreatment and emphasis on risk stratification among its main goals.[14] To illustrate, the 2015 guidelines no longer recommend fine needle aspiration (FNA) for high-risk nodules measuring <1 cm, invoking evidence of low disease-specific mortality, locoregional recurrence, and distant recurrence associated with papillary thyroid carcinoma less than 1 cm, referred to as papillary thyroid microcarcinoma (PTMC). Active surveillance is now recognized as an option even for biopsy-proven PTMC without concerning features such as cervical lymphadenopathy or evidence of extrathyroidal extension.[15] The "less is more" approach to treatment also manifests itself in the recommendations for the extent of thyroid surgery. Whereas the diagnosis of differentiated thyroid carcinoma historically mandated total thyroidectomy, thyroid lobectomy is now accepted as a valid option for select patients with a less than 4 cm papillary thyroid carcinoma.[11]

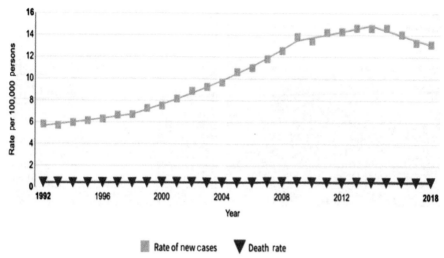

Fig. 2. Rate of new cases of thyroid cancer versus stable, low death rate from 1992 to 2018. (*From* SEER Cancer Stat Facts: Thyroid cancer. National Cancer Institute. Bethesda, MD, https://seer.cancer.gov/statfacts/html/thyro.html; with permission.)

Guidelines

Multiple societies have published guidelines for the management of thyroid nodules, including the American Thyroid Association (ATA), the American Association of Clinical Endocrinologists (AACE)/American College of Endocrinology (ACE)/Associazione Medici Endocrinologi (AME), and the British Thyroid Association (BTA). All guidelines recommend the use of ultrasound features to risk stratify nodules and guide management, although the ultrasound reporting systems vary between publications. The recommendation for follow-up ultrasound of benign nodules also varies among guidelines.

PATIENT EVALUATION
History and Physical

Evaluation of a patient with thyroid nodules begins with a thorough history, with particular attention to exposure to ionizing radiation, family history of thyroid cancer, and syndromes with an elevated risk of thyroid cancer, including Cowden disease, familial adenomatous polyposis, and multiple endocrine neoplasia type 2. Any history of rapid nodule growth or hoarseness ought to be elicited, though the majority of thyroid nodules are asymptomatic.[16] Physical examination should evaluate for the presence of a palpable, fixed nodule and cervical lymphadenopathy, although only 4% to 7% of patients have palpable nodules.[17]

Laboratories

Routine thyroid-stimulating hormone (TSH) should be obtained for all patients with a thyroid nodule greater than 1 cm.[14] An elevated TSH is associated with a higher risk of malignancy (ROM).[18] A low TSH should prompt further evaluation with a radionuclide scan to determine whether the nodule is hyperfunctional ("hot"), nonfunctional ("cold"), or isofunctional relative to the rest of the gland. Hyperfunctional nodules are less likely to harbor malignancy than cold nodules, but their ROM may be underestimated.[19] Cold nodules have a reported malignancy rate of 5% to 15%. However,

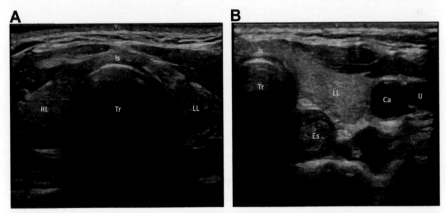

Fig. 3. (*A*) Ultrasound of normal thyroid gland. (*B*) Ultrasound of normal left thyroid lobe and surrounding normal anatomy. Ca, carotid artery; Es, esophagus; IJ, internal jugular vein; Is, isthmus; LL, left lobe; RL, right lobe; Tr, trachea.

the predictive value of a hypofunctioning nodule is low and specificity is lower in lesions less than 1 cm.[20] Serum thyroglobulin levels are nonspecific and are not a recommended component of thyroid nodule evaluation. Serum calcitonin measurement is not necessary for all patients, but may be appropriate in cases raising concern for medullary thyroid carcinoma (MTC), such as patients with a family history of MTC or patients with suspicious cytology not consistent with papillary thyroid carcinoma.[14]

Imaging

Ultrasonography is mandatory in patients with thyroid nodules. This modality is aptly suited to visualize and characterize thyroid nodules in a safe, comfortable, and efficient manner, without exposing a patient to radiation. Because of the thyroid gland's superficial location, high-resolution ultrasound provides excellent definition of the gland and any irregularities within it (**Fig. 3**).[21] Though CT and MRI can detect nodules, these modalities have not produced radiographic features that reliably correlate with benign or malignant disease.[22,23] Ultrasound, on the other hand, has a high sensitivity (96.1%) for identifying thyroid nodules that warrant biopsy because of its ability to delineate the features used to stratify them into risk categories: size, shape, consistency, echogenicity, border characteristics, and presence of microcalcifications.[24] In addition to evaluating the thyroid, ultrasound should also be used to evaluate the neck for any suspicious lymphadenopathy.

Ultrasound Reporting Systems

Ultrasound features of thyroid nodules allow for risk stratification and informed decision making regarding which nodules warrant biopsy. Multiple professional organizations have developed guidelines for reporting and risk stratification of thyroid nodules, including the American College of Radiology's Thyroid Imaging Reporting and Data System (ACR-TIRADS), the Korean Thyroid Imaging Reporting and Data System (K-TIRADS), the BTA, the European Thyroid Association Thyroid Imaging Reporting and Data System (EU-TIRADS), the AACE/ACE/AME, and the ATA. Though each society has adopted a slightly different approach to risk stratification, the intent is the same: to identify which thyroid nodules mandate further investigation and treatment, while minimizing the number of biopsies performed on benign nodules.[25]

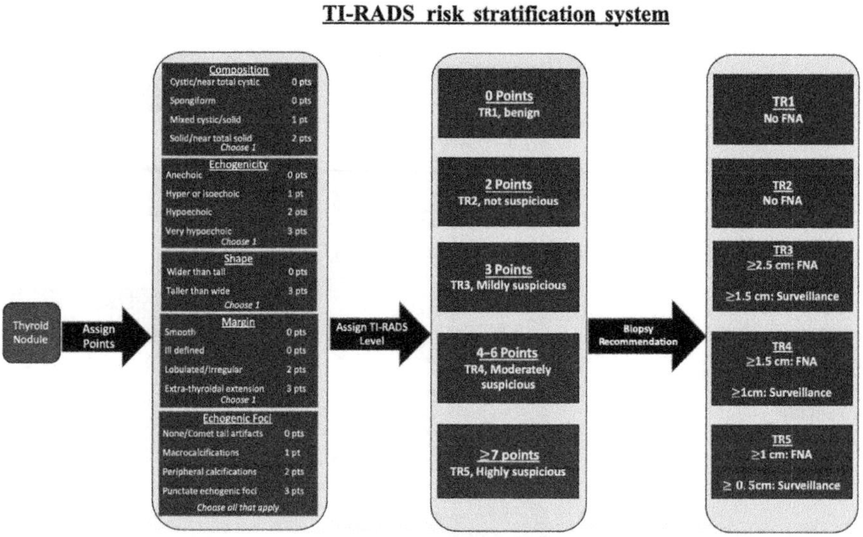

TI-RADS risk stratification system

Fig. 4. Depiction of the American College of Radiology TI-RADS ultrasonographic risk stratification system, which assigns points to a thyroid nodule based on the presence of suspicious features to categorize it into one of 5 TR categories, which in turn are used to inform recommendations for FNA and follow-up. (*Data from* ACR thyroid imaging, reporting and data system (TI-RADS): White paper of the ACR TI-RADS committee.)

The ACR-TIRADS system risk stratifies nodules by assigning points within 5 categories: composition, echogenicity, shape, margin, and echogenic foci (**Fig. 4**). Features within each category are assigned points based on their level of suspicion. One feature is selected from each of the first 4 categories, and all features that apply are selected from the echogenic foci category. The number of points assigned to the nodule determines its risk level, which ranges from TR1 (benign) to TR5 (high suspicion for malignancy). The nodule's TIRADS level and maximum diameter then determine recommendations for FNA or follow-up ultrasound. For TR3-TR5 nodules, FNA is recommended for a maximum diameter of ≥2.5 cm, ≥1.5 cm, and ≥1 cm, respectively.[25]

The ATA adopts a pattern-based approach that combines several sonographic features to classify a nodule into a risk category (**Fig. 5**). Internal consistency, shape, margin characteristics, echogenicity, and presence of microcalcifications are used to assign the nodule into one of five risk categories: benign, very low suspicion, low suspicion, intermediate suspicion, and high suspicion. Microcalcifications, irregular margins, and taller-than-wide shape are the features that most strongly correlate with thyroid cancer; a greater number of these features portends a higher ROM.[26,27] Taller-than-wide shape refers to an anterior-posterior dimension exceeding the transverse dimension when measured on an axial view.[14] Spongiform or purely cystic consistency, on the other hand, are features that are strongly associated with benignity.[14,28]

ATA High and Intermediate Suspicion Nodules

Nodules categorized as high suspicion are solid or partially solid, hypoechoic, and have one or more of the following features: microcalcifications, taller than wide shape, irregular margins, rim calcification disrupted by a solid hypoechoic component, or extrathyroidal extension (**Fig. 6**). The estimated rate of malignancy of a high suspicion nodule ranges from 70% to 90%.[14] Hypoechoic solid nodules without any additional

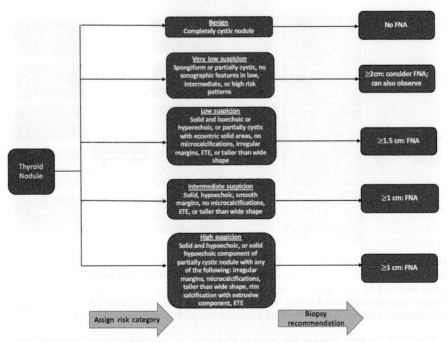

ATA risk stratification system

Fig. 5. Depiction of the American Thyroid Association pattern-based ultrasonographic risk stratification system, which assigns a nodule to a risk category based on a combination of ultrasound features and provides subsequent size criteria to guide recommendation for FNA. (*Data from* 2015 American Thyroid Association Management Guidelines for Adult Patients With Thyroid Nodules and Differentiated Thyroid Cancer: The American Thyroid Association Guidelines Task Force On Thyroid Nodules and Differentiated Thyroid Cancer.)

suspicious features are assigned to the intermediate-risk category, with an estimated malignancy risk of 10% to 20%.[14] FNA is recommended for high-risk and intermediate-risk nodules ≥1 cm.[14]

ATA Low and Very Low Suspicion Nodules

The low suspicion category includes isoechoic or hyperechoic nodules and partially cystic nodules with eccentric uniformly solid components, without any additional high-risk features. The estimated ROM for a low suspicion nodule is 5% to 10%, and FNA is not warranted unless the nodule measures ≥1.5 cm.[14] Very low suspicion nodules harbor a ≤3% ROM, and include spongiform and partially cystic nodules without any high-risk features (**Fig. 7**). Spongiform nodules are characterized by similarly sized microcystic spaces separated by thin, echogenic septae.[29] FNA can be offered for very low-risk nodules ≥2 cm, although observation is also a reasonable option.[14]

ATA Benign Nodules

Purely cystic nodules, characterized by a completely anechoic interior, are assigned to the benign category, for which FNA is not indicated (**Fig. 8**).[14]

It is important to note that guidelines, while providing an evidence-based framework for clinical decision making, are not absolute. A clinician's judgment and the patient's preferences and values should also influence the decision to perform FNA. For

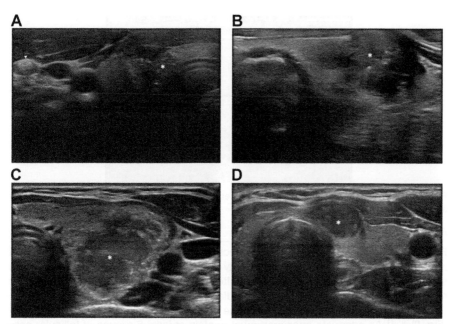

Fig. 6. Examples of ultrasonographic appearance of ATA high suspicion and intermediate suspicion nodules. (*A*) High suspicion hypoechoic nodule (*asterisk*) with irregular borders, microcalcifications, and extrathyroidal extension in the right superior lobe. A hyperechoic, rounded lymph node is visualized (*arrowhead*). (*B*) High suspicion hypoechoic nodule with irregular borders, microcalcifications, and extrathyroidal extension in the left thyroid lobe. (*C*) High suspicion hypoechoic nodule with taller than wide shape and irregular margins in the left thyroid lobe. (*D*) Intermediate suspicion solid hypoechoic nodule at the junction of the left isthmus and left superior lobe.

instance, it is appropriate to offer FNA at lower size cutoffs in patients with additional risk factors such as history of exposure to radiation or a family history of thyroid cancers. Likewise, surveillance can be offered as an alternative to FNA based on patient preference, high surgical risk, and shorter life expectancy.

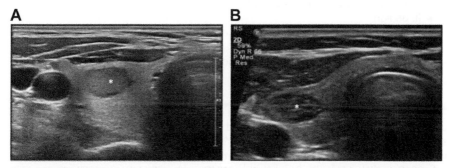

Fig. 7. Ultrasound examples of ATA low suspicion and very low suspicion nodules (*asterisks*). (*A*) Low suspicion, solid, isoechoic nodule without any suspicious features in the right thyroid lobe. (*B*) Very low suspicion spongiform nodule in the right thyroid lobe.

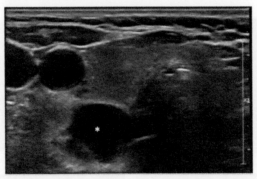

Fig. 8. Ultrasound appearance of an ATA benign, cystic nodule (*asterisk*), with a purely anechoic echogenicity.

Biopsy

FNA is the initially recommended biopsy technique endorsed by all major guidelines. It is well-tolerated, low risk, and technically simple enough to perform in the office setting. Core needle biopsy (CNB) is an alternative technique that may be useful for repeat biopsy in cases where FNA is nondiagnostic.

FNA performed with ultrasound guidance increases the rate of specimen adequacy (**Fig. 9**).[30,31] An adequate specimen must contain at least 6 groups of follicular cells containing 10 to 15 cells each (**Fig. 10**).[32] Immediate interpretation of cellular adequacy (performed by a pathologist or cytopathology technologist) decreases the rate of nondiagnostic specimens, especially when combined with ultrasound guidance.[30,33] The risks of FNA are low, with pain and minor hematomas being the most common.[34,35] Anticoagulant use does not appear to increase the risk of hematoma or inadequate cellularity.[36–38]

The Bethesda System

A standardized classification system for reporting thyroid FNA cytology results was proposed at the 2007 Thyroid Fine Needle State of the Art and Science Conference in Bethesda, Maryland. The Bethesda System for Reporting Thyroid Cytology (TBSRTC) is now the most widely used method for reporting thyroid nodule histology. The TBSRTC assigns a nodule to one of six categories, which in turn guide treatment options. Each category has a correlating ROM. The 6 categories are as follows:

- I: nondiagnostic or unsatisfactory
- II: benign
- III: atypia of undetermined significance (AUS) or follicular lesion of undetermined significance (FLUS)
- IV: follicular neoplasm (FN) or suspicious for a follicular neoplasm (SFN)
- V: suspicious for malignancy
- VI: malignant

FNA is highly sensitive for the detection of malignancy; a meta-analysis of 25,445 thyroid fine needle aspirations categorized with TBSRTC demonstrated a sensitivity, specificity, PPV, and NPV of 97%, 50.7% 55.9%, and 96.3%, respectively. The false-negative and false-positive rates were 3% and 0.5%, respectively.[39]

In 2016, the World Health Organization (WHO) reclassified the noninfiltrative encapsulated follicular variant of papillary thyroid carcinoma as "noninvasive follicular thyroid neoplasm with papillary-like nuclear features" (NIFTP).[40] This re-categorization

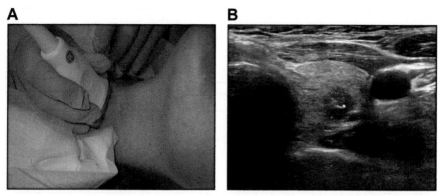

Fig. 9. Example of fine needle aspiration of left thyroid nodule. (*A*) The ultrasound probe is used to guide a 25 gauge needle on a 5 cc syringe into the thyroid nodule. The bevel of the needle is positioned superiorly toward the probe in order to better visualize the needle flash. (*B*) The tip of the needle (*) is visualized in the thyroid nodule on ultrasound.

subsequently decreased the previously estimated risks of ROM associated with each Bethesda category.[41] The associated ROM for each category is summarized below (**Table 1**), with and without NIFTP.

MANAGEMENT RECOMMENDATIONS

See **Fig. 11** for an algorithm depicting management of a thyroid nodule.

Management for Patients Who Undergo FNA

Patients who undergo FNA should be managed according to cytopathology results and the corresponding ROM.

Bethesda I (nondiagnostic)
Approximately 13% of FNA results are nondiagnostic.[39] Nodules with nondiagnostic cytology have a 1% to 4% predicted ROM.[42] A repeat FNA yields a diagnostic result

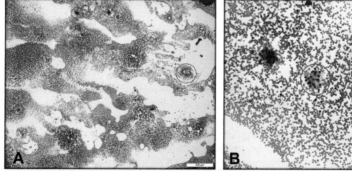

Fig. 10. Pathology slides from thyroid nodule FNA demonstrating appearance of follicular cells. (*A*) Slide at 4× magnification demonstrating 4 groups of follicular cells, circled in red. Additional groups were identified in other fields of the slide not captured in this image, therefore the FNA was deemed adequate by the pathologist. (*B*) 20× magnification of the same image demonstrating the appearance of a group of follicular cells counted toward the 6 groups necessary for an adequate specimen. The cells in the group have round to oval nuclei, are similar in size to each other, and have smooth nuclear borders.

Table 1 ROM for each Bethesda category			
Bethesda Category	**ROM (%) with NIFTP[a]**	**ROM (%) without NIFTP[b]**	**Management Options**
I Nondiagnostic	5%–10%	5%–10%	Repeat FNA vs core needle biopsy
II Benign	0%–3%	0%–3%	Clinical and radiologic follow-up
III Atypia of uncertain signification/follicular lesion uncertain significance	6%–18%	10%–30%	Repeat biopsy, molecular testing, surgery
IV Follicular neoplasm/suspicious for follicular neoplasm	10%–40%	25%–40%	Repeat biopsy, molecular testing, surgery
V Suspicious for malignancy	40%–60%	50%–75%	Surgery, active surveillance in select patients
VI Malignant	94%–95%	97%–99%	Surgery, active surveillance in select patients

[a] Risk of malignancy if the NIFTP category is used (ie, NIFTP nodules are not considered malignant).
[b] Risk of malignancy if the NIFTP category is not used (ie, NIFTP nodules are considered malignant).
   Cibas ES, Ali SZ. The 2017 bethesda system for reporting thyroid cytopathology. Thyroid. 2017;27(11):1341-1346.

in up to 80% of cases and should be performed.[43] Alternatively, CNB may also be offered. For nodules with repeatedly nondiagnostic cytology, sonographic features can guide decision making. Either observation or thyroid lobectomy for diagnostic purposes can be offered for a nodule without high-risk features. Surgery should be considered for histopathological diagnosis in cases of nondiagnostic nodules with suspicious sonographic features, in patients with clinical risk factors, or when growth of the nodule greater than 20% in 2 dimensions is detected during surveillance.[14]

Bethesda II (benign)
Benign nodules have a 0% to 3% ROM.[42] The recommended follow-up for thyroid nodules with benign cytology is determined by the ATA sonographic risk category, as described earlier (**Table 2**). Benign nodules with a high suspicion pattern warrant repeat ultrasound and FNA within 12 months. For nodules with a low to intermediate suspicion ultrasound pattern, repeat ultrasound can be performed in 12 to 24 months. Repeat FNA or continued surveillance with ultrasound should be offered if the nodule develops any new suspicious ultrasound characteristics, or if it demonstrates a 20% increase in 2 dimensions with a minimum increase of 2 mm or more than a 50% change in volume. Nodules with a very low suspicion ultrasound pattern do not require continued surveillance, and if ultrasound is repeated it should be performed no sooner than 2 years. Nodules that have undergone 2 FNAs with benign cytology have a negligible ROM and do not warrant additional follow-up.[27]

Bethesda III (AUS or FLUS) and Bethesda IV (FN or SFN)
Bethesda III and IV nodules are considered "indeterminate" and have a 6% to 40% ROM.[38] Treatment options include thyroid lobectomy for diagnostic purposes, continued surveillance, or repeat biopsy with addition of molecular testing if the

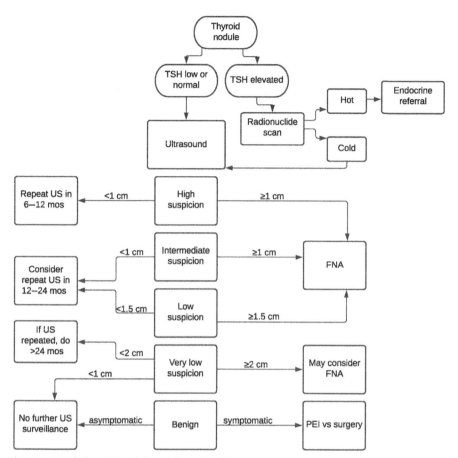

Fig. 11. Initial thyroid nodule workup algorithm.

cytology is again indeterminate. Clinical risk factors, sonographic pattern, and patient preference influence which of these options to choose. Performing a second FNA often yields diagnostic cytology, although up to 38.5% of nodules will again be categorized as AUS/FLUS.[44]

Bethesda V (suspicious for malignancy) and Bethesda VI (malignant)
Nodules with cytology consistent with malignancy or suspicious for malignancy generally warrant surgical management. Molecular testing may be considered if it is expected to alter surgical management. The extent of surgery (hemithyroidectomy vs total thyroidectomy) is discussed below.

PTMC surveillance option
In the era of de-escalation of thyroid cancer diagnostic and treatment intensity, active surveillance may be appropriate for low-risk PTMC without extrathyroidal extension or cervical lymphadenopathy.[15] Active surveillance protocols consist of ultrasounds every 6 months until no evidence of progression is observed over a 2-year period, at which point the surveillance interval can be increased to every 1 to 2 years. Surgery is reserved for cases that demonstrate increase in size, growth toward the thyroid capsule or adjacent structures, detection of nodal metastasis, or patient preference.[45]

Table 2
Recommended follow-up for thyroid nodules with benign cytology on FNA

Sonographic Pattern	Follow-up	Further Management
High suspicion (hypoechoic with irregular margins, microcalcifications, taller than wide, rim calcification with extrusive component, or ETE)	Repeat US and FNA within 12 mo	If second FNA is benign, no further follow-up is indicated
Intermediate suspicion (solid, hypoechoic, no additional features in high suspicion category) **Low suspicion** (solid and isoechoic or hyperechoic, or partially cystic with eccentric solid areas, no features in high suspicion category)	Repeat US in 12–14 mo	Repeat FNA or continued surveillance for: • New suspicious US characteristics • Growth ≥20% in 2 dimensions If stable size and no new suspicious features, no further follow-up indicated
Very low suspicion (spongiform or partially cystic, no additional features in low, intermediate, or high-risk categories)	No US surveillance is required; if offered, should be no sooner than 2 y	

This strategy is supported by PTMC's low disease-specific mortality (<1%) and indolent course.[46] In a series of 340 patients with PTMC undergoing active surveillance, the proportions of patients experiencing tumor growth greater than 3 mm were 6.4% and 15.9% at 5 and 10 years, whereas lymph node metastasis were detected in 1.4% and 3.4% at 5 and 10 years, respectively.[17] Moreover, patients who do undergo salvage surgery after an initial period of observation do not appear to suffer any greater morbidity or worse disease-related outcomes as a result of delayed surgery.[17,18]

Management for patients who do not undergo FNA
For nodules in which FNA is not indicated, the follow-up strategy is dictated by the sonographic risk category:

- High-suspicion nodules warrant repeat ultrasound in 6 to 12 months.
- Low to intermediate suspicion nodules should have an ultrasound in 12 to 24 mos.
- For very low suspicion or benign pattern nodules (ie, spongiform and purely cystic nodules) measuring >1 cm, the utility of continued surveillance is unclear. If repeat ultrasound is offered, it should be no sooner than 2 years. Follow-up is not indicated for low suspicion and purely cystic nodules measuring ≤1 cm.

Long-term recommendations
Current guidelines do not specify long-term recommendations for monitoring nodules that still do not meet indications for biopsy at the time of the initial follow-up ultrasound. The ideal follow-up duration and utility of repeat ultrasound in these cases are not clearly defined. Some guidelines recommend what amounts to a "massive

surveillance program," which is difficult to justify, considering that many of these nodules are incidentalomas.[47] Many practitioners recommend annual thyroid ultrasounds, although there is a lack of high-quality evidence to support this strategy. It is evident, however, that both physicians and patients are becoming aware of the "Pandora's box phenomenon," in which one test begets another without a clear benefit to the patient. As such, some investigators are identifying ways to decrease the risk of overtreatment.[47,48] One protocol suggests that in the absence of growth (>3 mm in any dimension) or concerning ultrasound features, routine annual ultrasounds after the initial follow-up ultrasound are not likely to be helpful and therefore recommends spacing out ultrasounds to every 2 to 3 years for a period of 5 to 10 years.[49] Lee and colleagues compared short-term and long-term follow-up of thyroid nodules with ultrasound and recommended against any follow-up beyond 3 years, as no meaningful changes in management occurred based on ultrasounds performed after 3 years. Long-term follow-up may result in multiple repeat FNA and ultrasounds without an improvement in the rate of cancer detection.[50]

Molecular testing

Thyroid nodule molecular testing is based on the principle that certain genetic alterations are associated with an increased ROM. It is indicated as an option for nodules with indeterminate FNA cytology, which occurs in approximately 20% to 30% of all thyroid FNAs. Molecular testing has the potential to decrease the number of unnecessary thyroid operations by ruling in or ruling out malignancy based on the identification of genetic alterations associated with malignancy.

The Afirma Gene Expression Classifier (GEC) test uses microarray technology to analyze mRNA expression of genes expressed in thyroid cancer. It was validated in a blinded prospective multicenter trial analyzing 265 indeterminate thyroid nodules from 4812 FNABs.[51] This study demonstrated an overall sensitivity of 92%, NPV of 93%, specificity of 52%, and PPV of 47%. The newest version of the Afirma test is the Gene Sequencing Classifier (GSC). A prospective blinded multi-institutional study evaluated the performance of the GSC on 191 Bethesda III/IV nodules with a cancer prevalence of 24%. The sensitivity, specificity, PPV, and NPV were 91%, 68%, 47%, and 96%, respectively.[52]

ThyroSeq is a next-generation sequencing (NGS) assay that analyzes DNA and RNA of thyroid-related genes for molecular alterations. ThyroSeq v3, the most current iteration, was validated in a prospective blinded cohort study involving 10 medical centers with analysis of 286 FNA samples from 1013 nodules. With respect to Bethesda III/IV nodules combined, the test demonstrated a 94% sensitivity and 82% specificity. The NPV and PPV were 97% and 66%, respectively, with a cancer prevalence of 28%.[53]

ThyGenX/ThyraMIR is a combined microRNA-based test. ThyGenX uses an NGS platform to identify more than 100 genetic alterations across 8 genes associated with thyroid malignancy. The ThyraMIR test is used as a reflexive test when the ThyGenX test is negative. A blinded multicenter cross-sectional cohort study of 109 Bethesda III/IV nodules from 638 FNAs evaluated the performance of the ThyGenX/ThyraMIR. Negative predictive value, PPV, sensitivity, and specificity were 94%, 74%, 89%, and 85%, respectively, with a cancer prevalence of 32%.[54] See **Table 3** for a summary of the main available molecular testing panels.

Further clarification is needed to determine the value of molecular testing in the management of thyroid nodules. Multiple studies demonstrate widely variable results compared with initial validation studies.[55–60] In addition, the accuracy of molecular testing platforms declines significantly when NIFTP reclassification is factored into

Table 3
Summary of the main commercially available molecular testing platforms

Panel	Afirma	ThyroSeq	ThyGenX/ThyraMIR
Mechanism	GEC: Analyze mRNA expression of 167 genes expressed in thyroid cancers. GSC: RNA sequencing evaluating >10,000 genes to detect point mutations, gene fusions, and copy number alterations	V3: Sequencing of 112 genes evaluating for mutations, rearrangements, gene expression alterations, and copy number variations	Combination of NGS panel of >100 genetic alterations across 8 genes (ThyGenX) and microRNA expression classifier (ThyraMIR) Starts with ThyGenX mutation analysis: if negative →reflexive ThyraMIR
Result reporting	Benign or suspicious	Test result: positive or negative Probability of cancer: low, medium, high Detailed result: specific genetic abnormalities	ThyGenX: specific gene mutations ThyraMIR: positive or negative

Abbreviations: GEC, gene expression classifier; GSC, genomic sequencing classifier; NGS, next-generation sequencing.

the initial validation studies.[59–61] Differences in study designs, lack of head-to-head comparisons, varying prevalence of malignancies in tested populations, and lack of final histologic data make results difficult to interpret and apply to the general population.[21,62,63] Until large cohort independent validation studies are available, molecular test results should be interpreted with caution.[21,62,63]

MEDICAL TREATMENT OPTIONS
Iodine

Patients with solid benign nodules should have adequate dietary iodine intake. If inadequate intake is detected or suspected, guidelines recommend consumption of a daily supplement containing 150 μg of iodine.[14]

Levothyroxine

TSH suppression with levothyroxine may modestly reduce thyroid nodule volume, but comes with the associated cost of hyperthyroidism, which may cause arrhythmias, bone loss, and other symptoms of thyrotoxicosis. Therefore, hormone suppression therapy is not routinely recommended for benign thyroid nodules.[14,64]

Radioactive Iodine

RAI may be used to treat toxic solitary nodules, toxic multinodular goiter (MNG), and nontoxic MNG in patients who are not candidates for surgery. Low doses of RAI have been shown to have durable effects on thyroid volume reduction and thyroid hormone normalization.[65–67]

SURGICAL TREATMENT OPTIONS

Surgical excision is the definitive treatment for any thyroid nodule. Surgery is recommended for nodules that are malignant or suspicious for malignancy, but may also be considered for indeterminate nodules in patients who do not desire continued surveillance or repeat biopsy. Surgery is also indicated for nodules that are compressive or otherwise symptomatic.

Extent of Thyroid Surgery

The extent of thyroid surgery (total vs hemithyroidectomy) is based on the presence of nodules in the contralateral lobe, the suspicion for malignancy, and patient preference. If there is a low likelihood of malignancy and the contralateral lobe is normal, a hemithyroidectomy is reasonable. Alternatively, a total thyroidectomy may be the preferred treatment option in the setting of suspicion for malignancy, particularly for bilateral nodules or a nodule that measures greater than 4 cm, shows signs of extrathyroidal extension, is suspect for aggressive histology, or has evidence of nodal spread. There has been a shift to more conservative thyroid surgery over the last decade, and current literature supports the appropriateness of hemithyroidectomy in cases of WDTC less than 4 cm with no adverse features.[68–70]

Risks of Thyroid Surgery

Risks specific to thyroid surgery include injury to the recurrent laryngeal nerve (RLN) and superior laryngeal nerve and hypoparathyroidism. The RLN innervates all intrinsic muscles of the larynx except the cricothyroid and should be identified in all thyroid surgery. The rates of temporary and permanent vocal cord weakness after thyroid surgery are approximately 10% and 2%, respectively.[71] The external branch of the superior laryngeal nerve (EBSLN) innervates the cricothyroid muscle. Injury to this nerve results in decreased vocal projection and pitch. This injury is difficult to quantify, and reported rates vary from 0% to 58%.[72–76] The parathyroid glands are located on the posterior aspect of the thyroid, near the inferior thyroid artery and RLN. Hypoparathyroidism and subsequent hypocalcemia may occur due to removal of the glands or disruption of their blood supply. Reported risks of temporary and permanent hypoparathyroidism are up to 32.8% and 12.5%, respectively.[77–80]

COMPLEMENTARY AND ALTERNATIVE TREATMENT OPTIONS

Options for minimally invasive management of thyroid nodules include image-guided thermal ablation (TA) and percutaneous ethanol injection (PEI).

Thermal Ablation

Image-guided TA includes radiofrequency ablation (RFA), laser thermal ablation (LTA), microwave ablation (MWA) and high-intensity focused ultrasound (HIFU). These modalities have the potential to decrease compressive symptoms and normalize suppressed thyroid hormone in properly selected patients. TA is an option for treating benign compressive nodules without high-risk US features.[81] Although no absolute size criteria are defined, a maximum diameter of 3 cm is suggested. TA may also be considered as a second-line treatment for autonomously functioning thyroid nodules (ATFN) after medical management or RAI. TA is not indicated for MNGs without a well-defined dominant nodule to target, or for Graves' disease or toxic MNG.

RFA and LTA are recommended as the first-line TA treatment modalities, with MWA considered a second-line option. HIFU is reserved for patients participating in clinical trials or who are unable to proceed with the other 3 options. A meta-analysis comparing the efficacy of RFA versus LTA for the treatment of 3195 solid benign nodules demonstrated a greater volume reduction with RFA compared with LTA at 6, 12, 24, and 36 months.[82,83] Efficacy for treating AFTN with TA is defined as restoration of normal thyroid function associated with a ≥80% reduction of initial volume. A meta-analysis reviewing RFA for autonomous nodules reported pooled rates of TSH normalization of 57%, scintigraphic cure rates of 60%, and volume reduction rates (VRRs) of 79% at 1 year.[84]

Ethanol

PEI is a particularly effective treatment for cystic nodules, whereas aspiration alone is associated with high (up to 80%) recurrence rates.[85] In a prospective randomized control trial, patients were randomized to undergo cyst aspiration (138 patients) or cyst aspiration plus PEI (143 patients). At 1-year post-treatment, volumes were decreased by 85.6% and 7.3% in the PEI and simple aspiration groups, respectively.[86] A systematic review including 1667 nodules demonstrated VRRs after PEI at 1, 2, 3, 5, and 10 years of 77%, 81%, 72%, 68%, 74%, and 69%.[87] PEI may also be considered for small (<5 mL volume) ATFN.[88]

COMPLICATIONS
Risks of Missing Thyroid Cancer or Delay in Diagnosis

The goal of managing thyroid nodules is to identify clinically significant malignancies without overtreating benign or clinically insignificant malignancies. One way of quantifying the complication of a "missed cancer" is to evaluate the outcomes of patients with a false negative benign FNA. In a retrospective review of 2010 benign FNA nodules, the false-negative rate was 1.3%.[89] Of the patients with a false-negative result, none died or had distant metastasis over an average follow-up of 11 years. Amit and colleagues reviewed 47 patients with false-negative FNA who underwent surgery at a mean of 52 months after biopsy. Five-year survival was 96%; multivariate analysis revealed that outcomes were not statistically different compared with patients who underwent immediate surgery for thyroid malignancy.[90] These results indicate that most clinically significant malignancies are identified on the first FNA and that initial benign cytology, even when later proven to be a false negative, tends to be associated with good long-term outcomes and low disease-specific mortality.

FUTURE DIRECTIONS

Important future directions include:

1. Improved differentiation between tumors with the potential to behave aggressively and become clinically significant versus tumors that will not result in any harm.

    To this end, additional components may ultimately be incorporated into risk stratification algorithms. For instance, nodule location has been reported to be an independent risk factor for thyroid cancer, with isthmus nodules portending the highest risk of cancer in a series of 3313 patients.[91] Further study is needed before additional features such as location become widely adopted in risk stratification systems for thyroid nodules.

    Furthermore, while active surveillance may be a reasonable option for PTMC, whether or not this strategy is appropriate for low-risk tumors greater than 1 cm remains to be determined. A recent study evaluated active surveillance in 291 patients with low-risk PTC up to 1.5 cm confined to the thyroid. Tumor growth was observed in 2.5% of patients at 2 years and 12.1% at 5 years, without any cases of regional or distant metastases. Notably, tumor size at presentation (<1 cm vs 1.0–1.5 cm) was not associated with tumor growth.[92] Additional studies regarding which patients with low-risk thyroid cancer can be offered surveillance, the safety of invoking salvage surgery as an option for patients whose disease does progress, and reporting of long-term

outcomes will be prerequisites to widespread implementation of active surveillance as an option for patients with WDTC.
2. A better understanding of the long-term efficacy of molecular testing and its ability to accurately predict which nodules require surgical intervention (and to what extent) versus which nodules can safely be observed.

Nodules with indeterminate cytology comprise 20% to 30% of thyroid nodules and remain a significant diagnostic challenge.[62] Incorporation of novel molecular markers will hopefully enhance the prognostic ability of molecular testing. Questions that remain to be answered and should be the emphasis of future research endeavors include whether or not molecular testing is guiding clinicians to avoid unnecessary surgeries, whether long-term follow-up for molecular marker negative nodules suggests a consistently indolent course, and whether molecular testing is a cost-effective strategy.
3. Greater consistency in ultrasound interpretation and reporting.

Methods to enhance the accuracy and reproducibility of ultrasound reporting are being explored. Ultrasound-based risk stratification is saturated with multiple systems, among which reporting is inconsistent, with a problematic amount of interobserver variability and overall subjectivity.[93] The multidisciplinary International Thyroid Ultrasound Working Group was recently formed with the aim of creating a unified international guideline that enhances consistency while reducing interobserver variability.[94]

As the management of thyroid nodules evolves, the goal of avoiding overtreatment must be balanced with caution to avoid undertreatment by demonstrating that patients who ultimately do harbor clinically significant disease are not harmed by any potential delay in treatment as a result of less aggressive screening and initial intervention.[86]

SUMMARY

Thyroid nodules are extremely common findings with a low likelihood of harboring a clinically significant malignancy. Clinical goals should be to identify malignancies while avoiding overtreatment and using a holistic, tailored approach to patients. The multiple published guidelines each recognize the importance of specific US characteristics in predicting malignancy. FNA should be performed based on US findings and risk categories and the Bethesda system should be used to classify FNA results. Molecular testing may be offered if the results are likely to change the therapeutic approach. Clinicians should be keenly aware of the potential for overtreatment and should make a concerted effort to factor patient values into the decision-making process.

CLINICS CARE POINTS

- Thyroid nodules are extremely common.
- Clinicians should be keenly aware of the potential for overtreatment of thyroid nodules and should make a concerted effort to factor patient values into the decision-making process.
- Ultrasound is the most important tool in the workup of thyroid nodules.
- High suspicion US features include hypoechogenicity, taller-than-wide shape, and microcalcifications.
- There are multiple different ultrasound classification systems with varying recommendations for size cut-off for FNA, but each one recognizes the risks associated with the above features.

- FNA cytology should be categorized using the Bethesda classification system.
- Molecular testing may be considered for indeterminate FNAs where the results would alter management.
- Further research is needed to improve the consistency of US reporting and the long-term implications of molecular testing.

DISCLOSURE

The authors have nothing to disclose.

REFERENCES

1. Jin J, McHenry CR. Thyroid incidentaloma. Best Pract Res Clin Endocrinol Metab 2012;26(1):83–96. https://doi.org/10.1016/j.beem.2011.06.004.
2. Mortensen JD, Woolner LB, Bennett WA. Gross and microscopic findings in clinically normal thyroid glands. J Clin Endocrinol Metab 1955;15(10):1270–80. https://doi.org/10.1210/jcem-15-10-1270.
3. Guth S, Theune U, Aberle J, et al. Very high prevalence of thyroid nodules detected by high frequency (13 MHz) ultrasound examination. Eur J Clin Invest 2009;39(8):699–706. https://doi.org/10.1111/j.1365-2362.2009.02162.x.
4. Ahmed S, Horton KM, Jeffrey RB Jr, et al. Incidental thyroid nodules on chest CT: review of the literature and management suggestions. AJR Am J Roentgenol 2010;195(5):1066–71. https://doi.org/10.2214/AJR.10.4506.
5. Rad MP, Zakavi SR, Layegh P, et al. Incidental thyroid abnormalities on carotid color doppler ultrasound: frequency and clinical significance. J Med Ultrasound 2015;23(1):25–8. Available at: https://www.sciencedirect.com/science/article/pii/S0929644114000769.
6. Yoon DY, Chang SK, Choi CS, et al. The prevalence and significance of incidental thyroid nodules identified on computed tomography. J Comput Assist Tomogr 2008;32(5):810–5. https://doi.org/10.1097/RCT.0b013e318157fd38.
7. Cohen MS, Arslan N, Dehdashti F, et al. Risk of malignancy in thyroid incidentalomas identified by fluorodeoxyglucose-positron emission tomography. Surgery 2001;130(6):941–6.
8. Desser TS, Kamaya A. Ultrasound of thyroid nodules. Neuroimaging Clin N Am 2008;18(3):463–78. https://doi.org/10.1016/j.nic.2008.03.005, vii.
9. Davies L, Welch HG. Current thyroid cancer trends in the United States. JAMA Otolaryngol Head Neck Surg 2014;140(4):317–22. https://doi.org/10.1001/jamaoto.2014.1.
10. Hoang JK, Nguyen XV, Davies L. Overdiagnosis of thyroid cancer: answers to five key questions. Acad Radiol 2015;22(8):1024–9.
11. Kovatch KJ, Hoban CW, Shuman AG. Thyroid cancer surgery guidelines in an era of de-escalation. Eur J Surg Oncol 2018;44(3):297–306.
12. US Preventive Services Task Force, Bibbins-Domingo K, Grossman DC, Curry SJ, et al. Screening for thyroid cancer: US preventive services task force recommendation statement. JAMA 2017;317(18):1882–7. https://doi.org/10.1001/jama.2017.4011.
13. Kim BW, Yousman W, Wong WX, et al. Less is more: comparing the 2015 and 2009 american thyroid association guidelines for thyroid nodules and cancer. Thyroid 2016;26(6):759–64. https://doi.org/10.1089/thy.2016.0068.

14. Haugen BR, Alexander EK, Bible KC, et al. 2015 american thyroid association management guidelines for adult patients with thyroid nodules and differentiated thyroid cancer: the American thyroid association guidelines task force on thyroid nodules and differentiated thyroid cancer. Thyroid 2016;26(1):1–133. https://doi.org/10.1089/thy.2015.0020.

15. Ramundo V, Sponziello M, Falcone R, et al. Low-risk papillary thyroid microcarcinoma: optimal management toward a more conservative approach. J Surg Oncol 2020;121(6):958–63. https://doi.org/10.1002/jso.25848.

16. Welker MJ, Orlov D. Thyroid nodules. Am Fam Physician 2003;67(3):559–66.

17. Popoveniuc G, Jonklaas J. Thyroid nodules. Med Clin North Am 2012;96(2): 329–49. https://doi.org/10.1016/j.mcna.2012.02.002.

18. Haymart MR, Repplinger DJ, Leverson GE, et al. Higher serum thyroid stimulating hormone level in thyroid nodule patients is associated with greater risks of differentiated thyroid cancer and advanced tumor stage. J Clin Endocrinol Metab 2008;93(3):809–14.

19. Lau LW, Ghaznavi S, Frolkis AD, et al. Malignancy risk of hyperfunctioning thyroid nodules compared with non-toxic nodules: systematic review and a meta-analysis. Thyroid Res 2021;14(1):3. https://doi.org/10.1186/s13044-021-00094-1.

20. Gharib H, Papini E. Thyroid nodules: clinical importance, assessment, and treatment. Endocrinol Metab Clin North Am 2007;36(3):707–35, vi.

21. Grani G, Sponziello M, Pecce V, et al. Contemporary thyroid nodule evaluation and management. J Clin Endocrinol Metab 2020;105(9):2869–83.

22. Nachiappan AC, Metwalli ZA, Hailey BS, et al. The thyroid: review of imaging features and biopsy techniques with radiologic-pathologic correlation. Radiographics 2014;34(2):276–93. https://doi.org/10.1148/rg.342135067.

23. Shetty SK, Maher MM, Hahn PF, et al. Significance of incidental thyroid lesions detected on CT: correlation among CT, sonography, and pathology. AJR Am J Roentgenol 2006;187(5):1349–56.

24. Hambly NM, Gonen M, Gerst SR, et al. Implementation of evidence-based guidelines for thyroid nodule biopsy: a model for establishment of practice standards. AJR Am J Roentgenol 2011;196(3):655–60. https://doi.org/10.2214/AJR.10.4577.

25. Tessler FN, Middleton WD, Grant EG, et al. ACR thyroid imaging, reporting and data system (TI-RADS): white paper of the ACR TI-RADS committee. J Am Coll Radiol 2017;14(5):587–95.

26. Salmaslioğlu A, Erbil Y, Dural C, et al. Predictive value of sonographic features in preoperative evaluation of malignant thyroid nodules in a multinodular goiter. World J Surg 2008;32(9):1948–54. https://doi.org/10.1007/s00268-008-9600-2.

27. Kwak JY, Han KH, Yoon JH, et al. Thyroid imaging reporting and data system for US features of nodules: a step in establishing better stratification of cancer risk. Radiology 2011;260(3):892–9. https://doi.org/10.1148/radiol.11110206.

28. Brito JP, Gionfriddo MR, Al Nofal A, et al. The accuracy of thyroid nodule ultrasound to predict thyroid cancer: systematic review and meta-analysis. J Clin Endocrinol Metab 2014;99(4):1253–63. https://doi.org/10.1210/jc.2013-2928.

29. Kim JY, Jung SL, Kim MK, et al. Differentiation of benign and malignant thyroid nodules based on the proportion of sponge-like areas on ultrasonography: Imaging-pathologic correlation. Ultrasonography 2015;34(4):304–11. https://doi.org/10.14366/usg.15016.

30. Redman R, Zalaznick H, Mazzaferri EL, et al. The impact of assessing specimen adequacy and number of needle passes for fine-needle aspiration biopsy of thyroid nodules. Thyroid 2006;16(1):55–60. https://doi.org/10.1089/thy.2006.16.55.

31. Robitschek J, Straub M, Wirtz E, et al. Diagnostic efficacy of surgeon-performed ultrasound-guided fine needle aspiration: a randomized controlled trial. Otolaryngol Head Neck Surg 2010;142(3):306–9. https://doi.org/10.1016/j.otohns.2009.11.011.

32. Gharib H, Goellner JR. Fine-needle aspiration biopsy of the thyroid: an appraisal. Ann Intern Med 1993;118(4):282–9. https://doi.org/10.7326/0003-4819-118-4-199302150-00007.

33. de Koster EJ, Kist JW, Vriens MR, et al. Thyroid ultrasound-guided fine-needle aspiration: the positive influence of on-site adequacy assessment and number of needle passes on diagnostic cytology rate. Acta Cytol 2016;60(1):39–45. https://doi.org/10.1159/000444917.

34. Polyzos SA, Anastasilakis AD. Clinical complications following thyroid fine-needle biopsy: a systematic review. Clin Endocrinol (Oxf) 2009;71(2):157–65. https://doi.org/10.1111/j.1365-2265.2009.03522.x.

35. Polyzos SA, Anastasilakis AD. A systematic review of cases reporting needle tract seeding following thyroid fine needle biopsy. World J Surg 2010;34(4):844–51. https://doi.org/10.1007/s00268-009-0362-2.

36. Denham SL, Ismail A, Bolus DN, et al. Effect of anticoagulation medication on the thyroid fine-needle aspiration pathologic diagnostic sufficiency rate. J Ultrasound Med 2016;35(1):43–8. https://doi.org/10.7863/ultra.15.03044.

37. Khadra H, Kholmatov R, Monlezun D, et al. Do anticoagulation medications increase the risk of haematoma in ultrasound-guided fine needle aspiration of thyroid lesions? Cytopathology 2018;29(6):565–8. https://doi.org/10.1111/cyt.12608.

38. Lyle MA, Dean DS. Ultrasound-guided fine-needle aspiration biopsy of thyroid nodules in patients taking novel oral anticoagulants. Thyroid 2015;25(4):373–6. https://doi.org/10.1089/thy.2014.0307.

39. Bongiovanni M, Spitale A, Faquin WC, et al. The bethesda system for reporting thyroid cytopathology: a meta-analysis. Acta Cytol 2012;56(4):333–9. https://doi.org/10.1159/000339959.

40. Nikiforov YE, Seethala RR, Tallini G, et al. Nomenclature revision for encapsulated follicular variant of papillary thyroid carcinoma: a paradigm shift to reduce overtreatment of indolent tumors. JAMA Oncol 2016;2(8):1023–9. https://doi.org/10.1001/jamaoncol.2016.0386.

41. Geramizadeh B, Maleki Z. Non-invasive follicular thyroid neoplasm with papillary-like nuclearfeatures (NIFTP): a review and update. Endocrine 2019;64(3):433–40. https://doi.org/10.1007/s12020-019-01887-z.

42. Cibas ES, Ali SZ. The 2017 bethesda system for reporting thyroid cytopathology. Thyroid 2017;27(11):1341–6. https://doi.org/10.1089/thy.2017.0500.

43. Saieg MA, Barbosa B, Nishi J, et al. The impact of repeat FNA in non-diagnostic and indeterminate thyroid nodules: a 5-year single-centre experience. Cytopathology 2018;29(2):196–200. https://doi.org/10.1111/cyt.12508.

44. Ho AS, Sarti EE, Jain KS, et al. Malignancy rate in thyroid nodules classified as bethesda category III (AUS/FLUS). Thyroid 2014;24(5):832–9. https://doi.org/10.1089/thy.2013.0317.

45. Brito JP, Ito Y, Miyauchi A, et al. A clinical framework to facilitate risk stratification when considering an active surveillance alternative to immediate biopsy and surgery in papillary microcarcinoma. Thyroid 2016;26(1):144–9. https://doi.org/10.1089/thy.2015.0178.

46. Mazzaferri EL. Management of low-risk differentiated thyroid cancer. Endocr Pract 2007;13(5):498–512.

47. Fradin JM. ACR TI-RADS: an advance in the management of thyroid nodules or pandora's box of surveillance? J Clin Ultrasound 2020;48(1):3–6. https://doi.org/10.1002/jcu.22772.

48. Jensen CB, Saucke MC, Francis DO, et al. From overdiagnosis to overtreatment of low-risk thyroid cancer: a thematic analysis of attitudes and beliefs of endocrinologists, surgeons, and patients. Thyroid 2020;30(5):696–703. https://doi.org/10.1089/thy.2019.0587.

49. Ajmal S, Rapoport S, Ramirez Batlle H, et al. The natural history of the benign thyroid nodule: what is the appropriate follow-up strategy? J Am Coll Surg 2015; 220(6):987–92.

50. Lee S, Skelton TS, Zheng F, et al. The biopsy-proven benign thyroid nodule: is long-term follow-up necessary? J Am Coll Surg 2013;217(1):81–9.

51. Alexander EK, Kennedy GC, Baloch ZW, et al. Preoperative diagnosis of benign thyroid nodules with indeterminate cytology. N Engl J Med 2012;367(8):705–15. https://doi.org/10.1056/NEJMoa1203208.

52. Endo M, Nabhan F, Porter K, et al. Afirma gene sequencing classifier compared with gene expression classifier in indeterminate thyroid nodules. Thyroid 2019; 29(8):1115–24. https://doi.org/10.1089/thy.2018.0733.

53. Steward DL, Carty SE, Sippel RS, et al. Performance of a multigene genomic classifier in thyroid nodules with indeterminate cytology: a prospective blinded multicenter study. JAMA Oncol 2019;5(2):204–12. https://doi.org/10.1001/jamaoncol.2018.4616.

54. Labourier E, Shifrin A, Busseniers AE, et al. Molecular testing for miRNA, mRNA, and DNA on fine-needle aspiration improves the preoperative diagnosis of thyroid nodules with indeterminate cytology. J Clin Endocrinol Metab 2015;100(7): 2743–50. https://doi.org/10.1210/jc.2015-1158.

55. Al-Qurayshi Z, Deniwar A, Thethi T, et al. Association of malignancy prevalence with test properties and performance of the gene expression classifier in indeterminate thyroid nodules. JAMA Otolaryngol Head Neck Surg 2017;143(4):403–8. https://doi.org/10.1001/jamaoto.2016.3526.

56. Baca SC, Wong KS, Strickland KC, et al. Qualifiers of atypia in the cytologic diagnosis of thyroid nodules are associated with different afirma gene expression classifier results and clinical outcomes. Cancer Cytopathol 2017;125(5): 313–22. https://doi.org/10.1002/cncy.21827.

57. Marcadis AR, Valderrabano P, Ho AS, et al. Interinstitutional variation in predictive value of the ThyroSeq v2 genomic classifier for cytologically indeterminate thyroid nodules. Surgery 2019;165(1):17–24.

58. Marti JL, Avadhani V, Donatelli LA, et al. Wide inter-institutional variation in performance of a molecular classifier for indeterminate thyroid nodules. Ann Surg Oncol 2015;22(12):3996–4001. https://doi.org/10.1245/s10434-015-4486-3.

59. Taye A, Gurciullo D, Miles BA, et al. Clinical performance of a next-generation sequencing assay (ThyroSeq v2) in the evaluation of indeterminate thyroid nodules. Surgery 2018;163(1):97–103.

60. Valderrabano P, Hallanger-Johnson JE, Thapa R, et al. Comparison of postmarketing findings vs the initial clinical validation findings of a thyroid nodule gene expression classifier: a systematic review and meta-analysis. JAMA Otolaryngol Head Neck Surg 2019;145(9):783–92. https://doi.org/10.1001/jamaoto.2019.1449.

61. Samulski TD, LiVolsi VA, Wong LQ, et al. Usage trends and performance characteristics of a "gene expression classifier" in the management of thyroid nodules: an institutional experience. Diagn Cytopathol 2016;44(11):867–73. https://doi.org/10.1002/dc.23559.

62. Khan TM, Zeiger MA. Thyroid nodule molecular testing: is it ready for prime time? Front Endocrinol (Lausanne) 2020;11:590128. https://doi.org/10.3389/fendo.2020.590128.

63. Singh Ospina N, Iñiguez-Ariza NM, Castro MR. Thyroid nodules: diagnostic evaluation based on thyroid cancer risk assessment. BMJ 2020;368:l6670. https://doi.org/10.1136/bmj.l6670.

64. Sdano MT, Falciglia M, Welge JA, et al. Efficacy of thyroid hormone suppression for benign thyroid nodules: meta-analysis of randomized trials. Otolaryngol Head Neck Surg 2005;133(3):391–6.

65. Nygaard B, Hegedüs L, Gervil M, et al. Radioiodine treatment of multinodular non-toxic goitre. BMJ 1993;307(6908):828–32. https://doi.org/10.1136/bmj.307.6908.828.

66. Roque C, Santos FS, Pilli T, et al. Long-term effects of radioiodine in toxic multinodular goiter: thyroid volume, function, and autoimmunity. J Clin Endocrinol Metab 2020;105(7):dgaa214. https://doi.org/10.1210/clinem/dgaa214.

67. Zingrillo M, Torlontano M, Ghiggi MR, et al. Radioiodine and percutaneous ethanol injection in the treatment of large toxic thyroid nodule: a long-term study. Thyroid 2000;10(11):985–9. https://doi.org/10.1089/thy.2000.10.985.

68. Haigh PI, Urbach DR, Rotstein LE. Extent of thyroidectomy is not a major determinant of survival in low- or high-risk papillary thyroid cancer. Ann Surg Oncol 2005;12(1):81–9. https://doi.org/10.1007/s10434-004-1165-1.

69. Adam MA, Pura J, Gu L, et al. Extent of surgery for papillary thyroid cancer is not associated with survival: an analysis of 61,775 patients. Ann Surg 2014;260(4):601–7. https://doi.org/10.1097/SLA.0000000000000925.

70. Nixon IJ, Ganly I, Patel SG, et al. Thyroid lobectomy for treatment of well differentiated intrathyroid malignancy. Surgery 2012;151(4):571–9. https://doi.org/10.1016/j.surg.2011.08.016.

71. Francis DO, Pearce EC, Ni S, et al. Epidemiology of vocal fold paralyses after total thyroidectomy for well-differentiated thyroid cancer in a medicare population. Otolaryngol Head Neck Surg 2014;150(4):548–57. https://doi.org/10.1177/0194599814521381.

72. Aluffi P, Policarpo M, Cherovac C, et al. Post-thyroidectomy superior laryngeal nerve injury. Eur Arch Otorhinolaryngol 2001;258(9):451–4. https://doi.org/10.1007/s004050100382.

73. Barczyński M, Randolph GW, Cernea CR, et al. External branch of the superior laryngeal nerve monitoring during thyroid and parathyroid surgery: international neural monitoring study group standards guideline statement. Laryngoscope 2013;123(Suppl 4):1. https://doi.org/10.1002/lary.24301.

74. Cernea CR, Ferraz AR, Furlani J, et al. Identification of the external branch of the superior laryngeal nerve during thyroidectomy. Am J Surg 1992;164(6):634–9.

75. Jansson S, Tisell LE, Hagne I, et al. Partial superior laryngeal nerve (SLN) lesions before and after thyroid surgery. World J Surg 1988;12(4):522–7. https://doi.org/10.1007/BF01655439.

76. Teitelbaum BJ, Wenig BL. Superior laryngeal nerve injury from thyroid surgery. Head Neck 1995;17(1):36–40. https://doi.org/10.1002/hed.2880170108.

77. Annebäck M, Hedberg J, Almquist M, et al. Risk of permanent hypoparathyroidism after total thyroidectomy for benign disease: a nationwide population-based cohort study from sweden. Ann Surg 2020. https://doi.org/10.1097/SLA.0000000000003800.

78. Cho JN, Park WS, Min SY. Predictors and risk factors of hypoparathyroidism after total thyroidectomy. Int J Surg 2016;34:47–52.

79. Ponce de León-Ballesteros G, Velázquez-Fernández D, Hernández-Calderón FJ, et al. Hypoparathyroidism after total thyroidectomy: importance of the intraoperative management of the parathyroid glands. World J Surg 2019;43(7):1728–35. https://doi.org/10.1007/s00268-019-04987-z.

80. Rosato L, Avenia N, Bernante P, et al. Complications of thyroid surgery: analysis of a multicentric study on 14,934 patients operated on in italy over 5 years. World J Surg 2004;28(3):271–6. https://doi.org/10.1007/s00268-003-6903-1.

81. Papini E, Monpeyssen H, Frasoldati A, et al. 2020 european thyroid association clinical practice guideline for the use of image-guided ablation in benign thyroid nodules. Eur Thyroid J 2020;9(4):172–85. https://doi.org/10.1159/000508484.

82. Ha EJ, Baek JH, Kim KW, et al. Comparative efficacy of radiofrequency and laser ablation for the treatment of benign thyroid nodules: systematic review including traditional pooling and bayesian network meta-analysis. J Clin Endocrinol Metab 2015;100(5):1903–11. https://doi.org/10.1210/jc.2014-4077.

83. Trimboli P, Castellana M, Sconfienza LM, et al. Efficacy of thermal ablation in benign non-functioning solid thyroid nodule: a systematic review and meta-analysis. Endocrine 2020;67(1):35–43. https://doi.org/10.1007/s12020-019-02019-3.

84. Cesareo R, Palermo A, Benvenuto D, et al. Efficacy of radiofrequency ablation in autonomous functioning thyroid nodules. A systematic review and meta-analysis. Rev Endocr Metab Disord 2019;20(1):37–44. https://doi.org/10.1007/s11154-019-09487-y.

85. Bennedbaek FN, Hegedüs L. Treatment of recurrent thyroid cysts with ethanol: a randomized double-blind controlled trial. J Clin Endocrinol Metab 2003;88(12):5773–7. https://doi.org/10.1210/jc.2003-031000.

86. Valcavi R, Frasoldati A. Ultrasound-guided percutaneous ethanol injection therapy in thyroid cystic nodules. Endocr Pract 2004;10(3):269–75.

87. Cesareo R, Tabacco G, Naciu AM, et al. Long-term efficacy and safety of percutaneous ethanol injection (PEI) in cystic thyroid nodules: a systematic review and meta-analysis. Clin Endocrinol (Oxf) 2021. https://doi.org/10.1111/cen.14530.

88. Guglielmi R, Pacella CM, Bianchini A, et al. Percutaneous ethanol injection treatment in benign thyroid lesions: role and efficacy. Thyroid 2004;14(2):125–31. https://doi.org/10.1089/105072504322880364.

89. Nou E, Kwong N, Alexander LK, et al. Determination of the optimal time interval for repeat evaluation after a benign thyroid nodule aspiration. J Clin Endocrinol Metab 2014;99(2):510–6. https://doi.org/10.1210/jc.2013-3160.

90. Amit M, Rudnicki Y, Binenbaum Y, et al. Defining the outcome of patients with delayed diagnosis of differentiated thyroid cancer. Laryngoscope 2014;124(12):2837–40. https://doi.org/10.1002/lary.24744.

91. Jasim S, Baranski TJ, Teefey SA, et al. Investigating the effect of thyroid nodule location on the risk of thyroid cancer. Thyroid 2020;30(3):401–7. https://doi.org/10.1089/thy.2019.0478.

92. Tuttle RM, Fagin JA, Minkowitz G, et al. Natural history and tumor volume kinetics of papillary thyroid cancers during active surveillance. JAMA Otolaryngol Head Neck Surg 2017;143(10):1015–20. https://doi.org/10.1001/jamaoto.2017.1442.

93. Persichetti A, Di Stasio E, Coccaro C, et al. Inter- and intraobserver agreement in the assessment of thyroid nodule ultrasound features and classification systems: a blinded multicenter study. Thyroid 2020;30(2):237–42. https://doi.org/10.1089/thy.2019.0360.

94. Tessler FN. Thyroid nodules and real estate: location matters. Thyroid 2020;30(3):349–50. https://doi.org/10.1089/thy.2020.0090.

Oral Cancer
What the General Surgeon Should Know

Cassie Pan, MD*, Zain Rizvi, MD

KEYWORDS

- Oral cavity cancer • Head and neck cancer • Squamous cell carcinoma

KEY POINTS

- The oral cavity consists of 7 subsites with distinct anatomic features. Knowledge of the unique characteristics of each subsite is essential in guiding the diagnostic and treatment approaches to oral cavity cancers.
- Tobacco and alcohol consumption are the dominant risk factors in the development of oral cavity cancer.
- Surgery is the mainstay of treatment of oral cavity cancers. The use of radiation therapy is limited by its extensive side effect profile in the oral cavity.

ANATOMY

The oral cavity represents a distinct anatomic region of the head and neck, with highly specialized functions in speech and expression, as well as deglutition and taste. It is bounded posteriorly by a coronal plane extending through the hard–soft palate junction and circumvallate papillae, and anteriorly by the vermillion border of the lips. Seven anatomic subsites of the oral cavity exist: lips, alveolar ridge (upper and lower), hard palate, anterior two-thirds of the tongue, floor of the mouth, retromolar trigone (RMT), and buccal mucosa (**Fig. 1**). These subsites have distinct anatomic characteristics as well as lymphatic drainage patterns (**Fig. 2**), leading to differences in the presentation, diagnosis, and treatment of tumors that arise from each subsite.

The lips form the orifice of the mouth, beginning anteriorly at the vermillion border and extending posteriorly to the labial sulcus. The orbicularis oris, a complex ring-like muscle underlying the lips, allows for sphincter contraction, providing oral competency for speech articulation and bolus retention during swallowing. The lips receive sensory innervation from trigeminal nerve branches and blood supply bilaterally from the labial arteries. Lymphatics from the upper lip typically drain to the ipsilateral

Department of Otolaryngology–Head and Neck Surgery, University of Washington, 1959 Northeast Pacific Street, Seattle, WA 98195, USA
* Corresponding author.
E-mail address: cpan1@uw.edu

Surg Clin N Am 102 (2022) 309–324
https://doi.org/10.1016/j.suc.2021.12.007
0039-6109/22/Published by Elsevier Inc.

surgical.theclinics.com

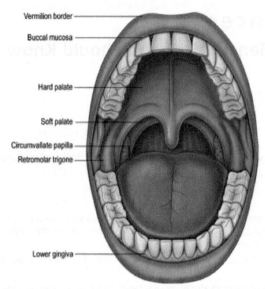

Fig. 1. Anatomy of the oral cavity. The oral cavity consists of 7 subsites with distinct anatomic characteristics and lymphatic drainage patterns. Subsites include lips, alveolar ridge (upper and lower), hard palate, anterior two-thirds of the tongue, floor of the mouth, retromolar trigone, and buccal mucosa. (*From* Andrew Foreman, Patrick J. Gullane. Overview of head and neck tumors. In: Plastic Surgery: Volume 3: Craniofacial, Head and Neck Surgery and Pediatric Plastic Surgery. Vol 3. 2nd ed. Elsevier Inc.; 2018:401-426.)

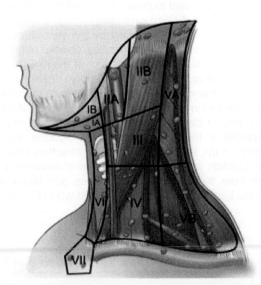

Fig. 2. Lymph node levels of the neck: IA, submental; IB, submandibular; IIA, upper jugular (anterior); IIB, upper jugular (posterior); III, mid jugular; IV, lower jugular; VA, upper posterior triangle; VB, lower posterior triangle; VI, pretracheal and paratracheal; VII, anterior mediastinal. (*From* Bryson TC, Shah GV, Srinivasan A, Mukherji SK. Cervical Lymph Node Evaluation and Diagnosis. Otolaryngologic Clinics of North America. 2012;45(6):1363-1383.)

submandibular, perifacial, and periparotid lymph nodes, while the lower lip drains to bilateral submandibular and submental triangles.

The alveolar ridge begins just posteriorly to the upper and lower labial sulci and is bounded laterally by the gingivobuccal sulci. Medially, the lower alveolus meets the floor of the mouth and the upper alveolus meets the hard palate. Each ridge consists of the tooth-bearing bone of the mandible and its tightly-adherent gingiva. Malignant tumors often demonstrate early cortical invasion via the closely approximated mucosa or medullary invasion via tooth roots, which extend into cortical bone. Sensory innervation is via the inferior alveolar branch of the mandibular nerve (V3), which travels through the mandible and exits at the mental foramen. Lymphatic drainage of anterior lesions involves submental and bilateral submandibular nodes while lateral lesions drain to ipsilateral submandibular and level II nodes.

The floor of the mouth extends from the medial lower alveolar ridge to the oral tongue and posteriorly to the anterior tonsillar pillars. It contains minor salivary glands, the sublingual glands, the submandibular ducts, as well as the lingual and hypoglossal nerves. Anterior lesions drain to levels IA and bilaterally to IB, whereas posterior and deep lesions tend to drain to ipsilateral level I and II nodes.

The anterior two-thirds of the tongue, or the portion anterior to the circumvallate papillae, defines the oral tongue subsite. This muscular structure has a highly innervated epithelium for sensation, supplied by the lingual nerve, and taste, supplied by the chorda tympani branch of the facial nerve. The mobility of the oral tongue, innervated by the hypoglossal nerve, is critical for articulation and deglutition. The tip primarily drains to level IA while lateral tongue lesions preferentially drain to ipsilateral levels I and II. Importantly, lateral tongue lesions can metastasize to levels III and IV even in the absence of level I and II disease.

The hard palate lies posterior and medial to the upper alveolar ridge and is bounded posteriorly by the soft palate. It consists of bone covered with tightly adherent mucosa with minor salivary glands. Important structures in the hard palate include the greater palatine, lesser palatine, and incisive foramen, which provide access for tumor spread. Sensory innervation is provided by the nasopharyngeal branch of the facial nerve. The hard palate preferentially drains to levels I and II and can also spread to retropharyngeal nodes.

The retromolar trigone is the triangular mucosal area that covers the ascending ramus of the mandible. It transitions to become buccal mucosa laterally and the anterior tonsillar pillar medially. As with the alveolar ridges, tumors in this area are prone to early mandibular invasion due to the closely adherent mucosa to the underlying bone. Sensation is supplied by the lesser palatine nerve (V2) and branches of the glossopharyngeal nerve. Lesions in the area may present with lower lip numbness due to the involvement of the nearby inferior alveolar nerve as it enters the mandibular foramen or referred otalgia due to the involvement of glossopharyngeal nerve branches. This subsite primarily drains to level II nodes.

Finally, the buccal mucosa represents the most lateral subsite of the oral cavity. It is bordered by the lips anteriorly, the alveolar ridges medially, and the RMT and pterygomandibular raphe posteriorly. Deep to the mucosa is the buccinator muscle, through which the parotid duct penetrates to terminate at Stenson's duct at the level of the second maxillary molar. The lack of bony confines and attachment of the pterygomandibular raphe to the pterygoid plate allows for the unopposed spread of buccal cancers and access to the skull base, respectively. Branches of the trigeminal nerve (V2 and V3) provide sensation to the buccal mucosa. Lymphatic drainage involves levels I and II and occasionally periparotid nodes.

EPIDEMIOLOGY

The oral cavity is the most common site of head and neck cancer. In 2020, it was the 11th most common malignancy in men and 18th most common malignancy in women worldwide.[1] Globally, oral cavity cancer was estimated to account for 380,000 new cancer cases in 2020, with a mortality rate of almost 50%.[1] The incidence of oral cavity cancer is 2.3 times greater in men than in women and also displays dramatic geographic differences.[1] Incidence is highest in Melanesia and South-Central Asia, whereby it approaches 10 per 100,000 people, compared with 4 to 5 per 100,000 people in the United States and countries of Western Europe (**Fig. 3**). In recent decades, the US incidence of oral cavity cancers has been decreasing, likely reflecting the decrease in smoking in the population.[2,3]

In addition to geographic and sex disparities, racial and socioeconomic status disparities also exist. In the US, black people with oral and oropharyngeal cancer have significantly worse overall and disease-specific survival rates and a 40% higher hazard of mortality compared with white people.[4] Furthermore, uninsured patients and those with low socioeconomic status have worse oral cavity cancer-specific survival than those with private insurance plans.[5,6]

The oral tongue and the floor of the mouth represent the 2 most common subsites and together account for more than half of all oral cavity cancers.[7,8] Greater than 90% of oral cavity tumors are squamous cell carcinomas (OSCC), followed by benign and malignant salivary gland tumors. Other uncommon tumors in the oral cavity include verrucous carcinoma, lymphoma, Kaposi's sarcoma, and mucosal melanoma. The wide diversity of tissue types in the oral cavity also leads to a variety of rare tumors, including osteosarcomas from bone, rhabdomyosarcomas from muscle, fibrosarcomas, and liposarcomas from other soft tissue, and nerve sheath tumors. The external lip is a subsite uniquely associated with sun exposure and can develop basal cell carcinoma and cutaneous melanoma and is considered separately from oral cavity cancers.

Incidence and Mortality Rates of Oral Cavity SCC by Geographic Region (2020)

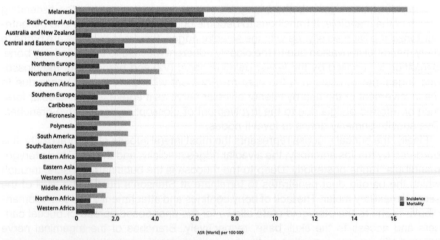

Fig. 3. The incidence and mortality rates of oral cavity squamous cell carcinoma differ by geographic region. ASR, age-standardized rate. (*Data from* Cancer today. Accessed June 19, 2021. http://gco.iarc.fr/today/home.)

ETIOLOGY

Tobacco and alcohol consumption are the most common risk factors associated with OSCC. Although these risk factors often occur together, each independently increases the risk of OSCC in a dose-dependent fashion.[9–11] Male smokers have an almost twofold greater risk of developing head and neck cancer compared with nonsmokers, and this risk increases in females.[12] Compared with nondrinkers, the risk of developing oral cancer is only marginally increased for light drinkers (≤1 drink per day), but almost five times greater in heavy drinkers (≥4 drinks per day).[12] Taken together, tobacco and alcohol act synergistically and contribute to an estimated 75% of all head and neck cancers.[13] This risk decreases with the cessation of tobacco and alcohol use and approximates the risk in nonusers after 20 years.[14–16]

OSCC can arise in patients with no history of tobacco and alcohol consumption, and the mechanism of carcinogenesis remains unclear. These nonsmokers and nondrinkers are more likely to be women and present at the extremes of age.[17,18] More recently, there has been a global trend of increasing incidence of oral tongue cancer in nonsmokers and nondrinkers under the age of 45, although the etiologic and clinical implications of this emerging group are not well-defined.[19–21] Other conditions that may rarely be associated with oral cavity cancers include chronic mucosal trauma such as bite trauma or poorly fitting dentures, long-term immunosuppression, and HIV infection.[22,23]

In certain parts of the world, including Southeast Asia and the Pacific Islands, betel nut is an important risk factor for the development of oral cavity cancer and likely accounts for the significantly higher incidence in these populations.[1] It is often crushed, mixed with lime, spices, and sometimes tobacco, and chewed as betel quid, which is an independent carcinogen even without the addition of tobacco (**Fig. 4**).[24,25]

Recent attention has been given to the role that high-risk HPV may play in oncogenesis in OSCC. Unlike in oropharyngeal cancers, whereby HPV-positive tumors are known to have unique epidemiologic, molecular, biologic, and prognostic differences compared with HPV-negative tumors, no clear etiologic role for HPV has been shown

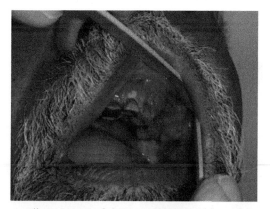

Fig. 4. Oral squamous cell carcinoma of the upper alveolar ridge, often associated with the chewing of betel quid. (*From* Andrew Foreman, Patrick J. Gullane. Overview of head and neck tumors. In: Plastic Surgery: Volume 3: Craniofacial, Head and Neck Surgery and Pediatric Plastic Surgery. Vol 3. 2nd ed. Elsevier Inc.; 2018:401-426.)

in OSCCs.[26] Thus, current guidelines for oral cavity cancers do not include HPV testing as it has not been shown to alter clinical course or treatment recommendations.

DIAGNOSIS AND EVALUATION

Oral malignancies present in a wide variety of forms, from a small irregular mucosal patch to a large fungating mass. Oral leukoplakia, a white patch or plaque that cannot be rubbed off, is associated with chronic irritation and smoking and has a 5% to 20% risk of malignant transformation[27,28] (**Fig. 5A**). Close monitoring of leukoplakia is recommended, and biopsy should be considered at initial presentation or with any clinical changes. In contrast, erythroplakia, or red patches or plaques, has a higher malignant potential and mandates biopsy[29–31] (**Fig. 5B**).

Patients may complain of nonhealing ulcers, persistent pain, halitosis, or bleeding without antecedent trauma. Other concerning signs and symptoms may indicate more advanced disease with the involvement of certain structures. These may include otalgia, trismus, loose teeth, changes in the fit of dentures, facial numbness, weight loss, dysarthria, dysphagia, and odynophagia. A thorough history should include medical comorbidities and medications, tobacco and alcohol use history, as well as prior surgeries.

Physical examination consisting of a complete head and neck examination, including cranial nerves, is key. As patients with oral cavity cancer often have the same risk factors for oropharyngeal, hypopharyngeal, and laryngeal cancers, these areas should be thoroughly evaluated using a mirror examination or flexible laryngoscopy to rule out a second primary. Regarding the oral cavity lesion, the examiner should specifically note the lesion's dimensions, depth, and mobility, involved subsites of the oral cavity and oropharynx, midline extension, and presence of any palpable regional lymphadenopathy. Assessment of local, regional, and distant donor sites for reconstructive potential is also important for surgical planning.

Tissue pathologic diagnosis remains the gold standard; thus the decision to biopsy a lesion depends on the patient's individual risk factors and the surgeon's clinical suspicion. Oral cavity lesions and suspicious neck lymphadenopathy are usually accessible for biopsy or fine-needle aspiration under local anesthesia in the clinic. Tumor biopsy should be aimed at obtaining a sample of adequate viability and depth for pathologic diagnosis and staging.

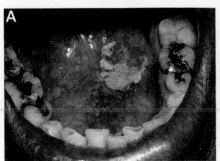 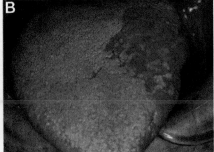

Fig. 5. (A) Leukoplakia of floor of the mouth. (B) Erythroplakia of lateral tongue. (*Adapted from* Joseph A. Regezi, James J. Sciubba, Richard C.K. Jordan. Oral Pathology. 7th ed. Elsevier Inc.; 2017.)

Imaging is used to further characterize the primary lesion, evaluate for regional and distant metastasis, and aid in treatment planning. Standard evaluation includes CT or MRI of the neck as well as a CT of the chest to evaluate for distant metastatic disease. Plain films have limited utility in evaluating oral cavity lesions. MRI is preferred for evaluating soft tissue invasion, extension into medullary bone, and nerve involvement. Contrast-enhanced CT is currently the most widely used modality for evaluating oral cavity cancer and has the advantage over MRI for demonstrating bony involvement (**Fig. 6**).

Accurately evaluating for bony involvement is critical in subsites with early bony invasion, including the RMT, alveolar ridge, and hard palate. Unfortunately, in these high-risk areas, early invasion may not be appreciated on any imaging modality and may only be detected on final pathology. As such, careful clinical examination is necessary and resection including bone may be required if occult bony invasion is suspected. With recent advancements in technology, PET and PET-CT have gained popularity, but their role in the evaluation of oral cavity cancer has not yet become standardized. PET has poor anatomic resolution and thus has major limitations in the evaluation of oral cavity tumors.[32] Even with combined PET-CT, the limited spatial resolution and dental artifacts make it inadequate for the imaging of small and superficial primary lesions.[33,34] For the assessment of cervical metastasis, CT and MRI offer similar diagnostic sensitivity, and data on the accuracy of PET-CT are evolving.[35] However, PET-CT has shown good diagnostic sensitivity for detecting distant metastases in patients with head and neck cancer.[36]

STAGING AND PROGNOSIS

Staging for oral cavity cancer follows the TNM staging format as defined by the American Joint Committee on Cancer (AJCC) 8th Edition (**Figs 7** and **8**). Recent updates improve prognostic stratification and importantly, incorporate the depth of invasion (DOI) in T-stage, which is directly correlated with the risk of nodal metastasis and portends a negative prognosis.[37–40] However, it does not account for additional tumor characteristics of prognostic importance. Tumors with smooth, well-defined, or

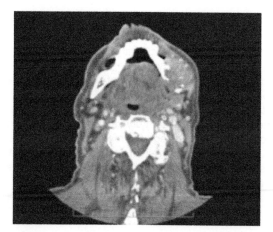

Fig. 6. Axial CT scan showing mandibular cancer with the erosion of bone. (*From* Andrew Foreman, Patrick J. Gullane. Overview of head and neck tumors. In: Plastic Surgery: Volume 3: Craniofacial, Head and Neck Surgery and Pediatric Plastic Surgery. Vol 3. 2nd ed. Elsevier Inc.; 2018:401-426.)

Primary Tumor (T)	
Tx	Primary tumor cannot be assessed
Tis	Carcinoma *in situ*
T1	Tumor ≤2 cm with DOI ≤5 mm
T2	Tumor ≤2 cm with DOI >5 mm *or*
	tumor >2 cm and ≤4 cm, with DOI ≤10 mm
T3	Tumor >2 cm and ≤4 cm, with DOI >10 mm *or*
	tumor >4 cm with DOI ≤10 mm
T4a	Moderately advanced local disease
	Tumor >4 cm with DOI >10 mm *or*
Lip	Tumor invades cortical bone or involves inferior alveolar nerve, FOM, or skin of face
Oral cavity	Tumor invades adjacent structures only (i.e. cortical bone of mandible or maxilla, maxillary sinus, or skin of face)
	Note: *superficial erosion of bone/tooth socket (alone) by gingival primary is not sufficient to classify as T4*
T4b	Very advanced local disease
	Tumor invades masticator space, pterygoid plates, or skull base and/or encases internal carotid artery
Regional Lymph Nodes (N)	
NX	Regional lymph nodes cannot be assessed
c/p N0	No regional lymph node metastasis
c/p N1	Metastasis in single ipsilateral lymph node, ≤3 cm in greatest dimension, ENE(-)
c/p N2a	Metastasis in single ipsilateral lymph node, >3 cm and ≤6 cm in greatest dimension, ENE(-) or
pN2a	Metastasis in single ipsilateral lymph node, ≤3 cm in greatest dimension and ENE(+)
c/p N2b	Metastasis in multiple ipsilateral lymph nodes, ≤6 cm in greatest dimension, ENE(-)
c/p N2c	Metastasis in bilateral or contralateral lymph nodes, ≤6 cm in greatest dimension, ENE(-)
c/p N3a	Metastasis in lymph node >6 cm in greatest dimension
N3b	
cN3b	Metastasis in any node(s) and clinically overt ENE(+)
pN3b	Metastasis in single ipsilateral node >3 cm in greatest dimension and ENE(+); or multiple ipsilateral, contralateral or bilateral nodes with ENE(+); or single contralateral node with ENE(+)
Distant Metastasis (M)	
M0	No distant metastasis
M1	Distant metastasis

DOI, depth of invasion; FOM, floor of mouth; ENE, extranodal extension.

Fig. 7. ENE, extranodal extension. *Data from* Keung EZ, Gershenwald JE. The eighth edition American Joint Committee on Cancer (AJCC) melanoma staging system: implications for melanoma treatment and care, Expert Review of Anticancer Therapy 2018;18(8):775-784.

"pushing" borders have improved prognosis compared with infiltrative tumors with less defined borders.[41] Conversely, perineural invasion is associated with significantly decreased overall and disease-free survival.[42] Additional variables that have been found to be independent prognostic factors of overall survival in oral cavity SCC include age, comorbidities, and vascular invasion.[42]

The most important prognostic factor in oral cavity cancer is the presence of cervical lymph node metastasis. The 5-year survival rate for localized disease is greater than 80% and drops to 50% with regional metastasis and to less than 30% with distant metastasis.[43] Furthermore, burden of neck disease is a negative prognostic indicator, as patients with a higher proportion of positive cervical nodes have increased risk of recurrence and decreased survival.[44]

TREATMENT

Treatment recommendations for oral cavity cancer follow the guidelines outlined by the National Comprehensive Care Network Clinical Practice Guidelines for Head and Neck Cancers, which are currently based on the AJCC 8th Edition staging

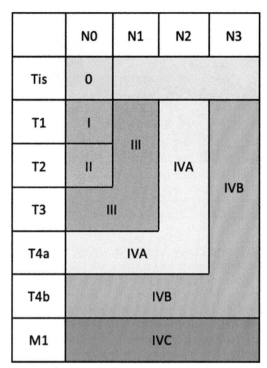

	N0	N1	N2	N3
Tis	0			
T1	I	III	IVA	IVB
T2	II		IVA	IVB
T3	III			IVB
T4a	IVA			
T4b	IVB			
M1	IVC			

Fig. 8. Prognostic stage groups based on AJCC 8th Edition TNM Staging. *Data from* Keung EZ, Gershenwald JE. The eighth edition American Joint Committee on Cancer (AJCC) melanoma staging system: implications for melanoma treatment and care, Expert Review of Anticancer Therapy 2018;18(8):775-784.

system.[45] Early-stage oral cavity cancers are generally treated with primary surgery or definitive radiation, whereas advanced-stage tumors often require multimodality treatment. While guidelines are based on the stage of disease and tumor characteristics, finding the optimal treatment of a patient necessitates an informed discussion of options and shared decision making, considering each patient's comorbidities, preferences, and goals of care.

Surgery

Primary surgical resection is the mainstay of the management of oral cavity malignancies. Surgery provides excellent oncologic outcomes for early stage tumors and is used for primary disease control in advanced-stage tumors, usually with adjuvant radiation therapy with or without chemotherapy. Additionally, surgery allows for accurate staging and histopathologic characterization of the tumor, including the presence of aggressive features that may warrant adjuvant treatment. Small tumors (T1s and select T2s) can usually be resected transorally (**Fig. 9**). Larger tumors and tumors with posterior extension toward the base of the tongue may require alternate techniques to achieve access, including mandibulotomy or transoral robotic-assisted surgery. Surgical resection and reconstruction of each subsite in the oral cavity require unique functional considerations related to speech, swallowing, breathing, taste, and smell, which should be managed without compromising the oncologic resection.

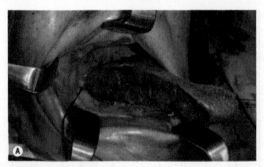

Fig. 9. Transoral approach with adequate retraction is often sufficient for accessing the anterior two-thirds of the tongue. (*From* Andrew Foreman, Patrick J. Gullane. Overview of head and neck tumors. In: Plastic Surgery: Volume 3: Craniofacial, Head and Neck Surgery and Pediatric Plastic Surgery. Vol 3. 2nd ed. Elsevier Inc.; 2018:401-426)

In surgical planning for oral cavity cancers, especially for more advanced tumors, it is essential to consider the impact that surgery will have on the patient's airway, as well as on speech and swallowing. Temporary tracheostomy may be required for large posterior reconstructions if there is concern that postoperative edema may impact airway patency. Alternate means of nutrition must also be explored, often with a nasogastric or gastrostomy tube, if the patient will be kept *nil per os* postoperatively or if swallowing difficulties, temporary or permanent, are anticipated based on the extent of resection and comorbidities. In patients undergoing free flap reconstruction, a prior history of radiation, volume of base of the tongue resected, and integrity of hypoglossal nerve were predictive of postoperative dysphagia.[46] For both speech and swallow impairments, early engagement with Speech and Language Pathology is an important resource to familiarize patients with alternate communication strategies, swallow therapy, and ease their postsurgical rehabilitation.

The primary goal of surgical resection is to remove all tumor cells. The gold standard for evaluating the completeness of resection is the assessment of margin status on permanent pathology. Positive margins are associated with poor prognosis and increased risk of local recurrence.[47–49] Assessment of margins intraoperatively currently relies on the surgeon's clinical judgment through visualization and palpation. Frozen section analysis is standard practice for intraoperative margin assessment, but is time-intensive, costly, prone to inconsistencies, and most importantly has not been shown to favorably impact local control or survival.[50–53]

In addition to the surgical resection of the primary lesion, surgical management of the neck must be considered. Treatment of clinically, radiographically, or biopsy-positive neck disease typically involves modified radical neck dissection (with the preservation of the spinal accessory nerve, internal jugular vein, and sternocleidomastoid muscle) of the involved or at-risk nodal levels. More advanced neck disease with the involvement of structures like the spinal accessory nerve or jugular vein may require the sacrifice of additional structures and lead to increased morbidity. Surgical management of the N0 neck in early-stage oral cavity cancer has long been controversial. Current guidelines note only low-to-moderate quality evidence for elective neck dissection (END) in node-negative early stage cancer and make no stronger recommendation than to "offer" an END to patients in these cases.[54,55] Recently, however, evidence is emerging that END improves overall and disease-free survival regardless of tumor size, and thus more surgeons are advocating for END even in small tumors without evidence of nodal disease.[56,57] DOI has proven to be an important guide in deciding when to perform END, with improved survival and local recurrence rates after END for DOI $\geq$4 mm.[58,59]

Reconstruction after ablative surgery is aimed at restoring form and function, particularly regarding speech and swallow. Defects from early stage tumors can often be primarily closed or reconstructed with a skin graft or local flap with little impact on functional outcome. Reconstruction of larger defects typically requires the expertise of an experienced head and neck reconstructive surgeon who can perform microvascular free tissue transfer. Commonly used free flaps in oral reconstruction include the radial forearm free flap, which is an excellent option for the soft tissue reconstruction of the tongue, floor of the mouth, and RMT, and the fibula free flap, which is well-suited to the bony reconstruction of segmental mandibulectomy.

Radiation Therapy

Radiation therapy remains a key treatment component for oral cavity cancers. Though surgery remains the gold standard of treatment, primary radiation therapy can be used to treat early-stage oral cavity cancer. When used as definitive treatment, it is typically given at a total dose of 66 to 70 Gy at 2.0 to 2.2 Gy/fraction over 6 to 7 weeks.[54] Adjuvant radiation after surgical resection is usually given at a lower dose and is indicated for multiple positive nodes, extranodal extension, positive or close margins, perineural invasion, lymphovascular invasion, and T3 or T4 primaries.[54] The extensive side effect profile of radiation treatment to the oral cavity favors surgery as the primary modality for the treatment of oral cavity cancer. Complications include xerostomia, mucositis, dental caries, tissue fibrosis, and in the context of neck irradiation, atherosclerosis. For the oral cavity, the most feared complication is osteoradionecrosis (ORN) of the mandible, which can lead to secondary infections, problems maintaining adequate nutrition, pathologic fracture, and need for further surgical intervention.

Chemotherapy

The role of chemotherapy in the definitive treatment setting remains limited to postoperative adjuvant treatment along with radiation therapy if extracapsular extension is present in nodal disease. It is also sometimes used in locally very advanced disease or if other adverse features like perineural or vascular invasion are present, but the evidence to support these indications is less robust.[54] Standard chemotherapy regimens used in the head and neck include platinum-based agents, with significant side effect profiles including neurotoxicity, ototoxicity, and renal impairment. In recent years, several studies have examined the safety and efficacy of definitive chemoradiation for locally advanced oral cavity SCC for organ preservation, but the risk of ORN with primary chemoradiation remains a concern and more data are needed before this treatment can be widely recommended.[60–62] Systemic therapy is also indicated for recurrent and metastatic disease not amenable to surgery or radiation, often involving PD-1 inhibitors or EGFR inhibitors used alone or in combination with platinated agents.

Surveillance

The majority of recurrences after treatment of oral cancer occur in the first 2 years.[63,64] Follow-up involves a complete history and head and neck examination (including mirror or fiberoptic examination) every 1 to 3 months for the first year, every 2 to 6 months for the second year, gradually spacing out the interval until 5 years posttreatment.[54] The surveillance plan should be adjusted based on patient-specific factors including risk of relapse, second primaries, need for supportive care, and monitoring of treatment complications. Routine use of surveillance imaging remains unstandardized, but is generally recommended within 3 to 4 months after definitive treatment for locoregionally advanced disease or with altered anatomy that makes physical examination challenging to establish a baseline for subsequent comparisons.[54]

CLINICS CARE POINTS

- Patients with suspected oral cavity cancer require a full head and neck physical examination including cranial nerves and mirror examination or flexible laryngoscopy to evaluate the oropharynx, hypopharynx, and larynx for a second primary.

- Close monitoring of oral leukoplakia is recommended, and biopsy should be considered at initial presentation or with any clinical changes. In contrast, oral erythroplakia has a high malignant potential and mandates biopsy.

- Imaging for oral cavity cancer should be obtained to characterize the primary lesion and evaluate for regional and distant metastatic disease. Typically, CT or MRI of the neck and CT of the chest are used.

- In surgical planning, impact on speech, swallow, and airway must be considered and planned for accordingly (ie, with use of nasogastric tube, gastrostomy tube, tracheostomy).

- Monitoring of side effects after radiation therapy to the oral cavity is essential, as complications can be extensive and lead to chronic medical problems.

DISCLOSURE

Funding/support: This work was supported in part by the grant T32DC000018 from the National Institutes of Health (Dr. Pan)

REFERENCES

1. Cancer today. Available at: http://gco.iarc.fr/today/home. Accessed June 19, 2021.
2. Carvalho AL, Nishimoto IN, Califano JA, et al. Trends in incidence and prognosis for head and neck cancer in the United States: A site-specific analysis of the SEER database. Int J Cancer 2005;114(5):806–16.
3. Weatherspoon DJ, Chattopadhyay A, Boroumand S, et al. Oral cavity and oropharyngeal cancer incidence trends and disparities in the United States: 2000–2010. Cancer Epidemiol 2015;39(4):497–504.
4. Osazuwa-Peters N, Massa ST, Christopher KM, et al. Race and sex disparities in long-term survival of oral and oropharyngeal cancer in the United States. J Cancer Res Clin Oncol 2016;142(2):521–8.
5. Kwok J, Langevin SM, Argiris A, et al. The impact of health insurance status on the survival of patients with head and neck cancer. Cancer 2010;116(2):476–85.
6. Agarwal P, Agrawal RR, Jones EA, et al. Social Determinants of Health and Oral Cavity Cancer Treatment and Survival: A Competing Risk Analysis. Laryngoscope 2020;130(9):2160–5.
7. SEER cancer Statistics Review 1975-2008 - Previous Version - SEER cancer Statistics. SEER. Available at: https://seer.cancer.gov/archive/csr/1975_2008/index.html. Accessed July 6, 2021.

8. Farhood Z, Simpson M, Ward GM, et al. Does anatomic subsite influence oral cavity cancer mortality? A SEER database analysis. The Laryngoscope 2019; 129(6):1400–6.

9. Hashibe M, Brennan P, Benhamou S, et al. Alcohol drinking in never users of tobacco, cigarette smoking in never drinkers, and the risk of head and neck cancer: pooled analysis in the International Head and Neck Cancer Epidemiology Consortium. J Natl Cancer Inst 2007;99(10):777–89.

10. Znaor A, Brennan P, Gajalakshmi V, et al. Independent and combined effects of tobacco smoking, chewing and alcohol drinking on the risk of oral, pharyngeal and esophageal cancers in Indian men. Int J Cancer 2003;105(5):681–6.

11. Ng SKC, Kabat GC, Wynder EL. Oral Cavity Cancer in Non-Users of Tobacco. J Natl Cancer Inst 1993;85(9):743–5.

12. Turati F, Garavello W, Tramacere I, et al. A meta-analysis of alcohol drinking and oral and pharyngeal cancers. Part 2: results by subsites. Oral Oncol 2010;46(10): 720–6.

13. Blot WJ, McLaughlin JK, Winn DM, et al. Smoking and drinking in relation to oral and pharyngeal cancer. Cancer Res 1988;48(11):3282–7.

14. Macfarlane GJ, Zheng T, Marshall JR, et al. Alcohol, tobacco, diet and the risk of oral cancer: a pooled analysis of three case-control studies. Eur J Cancer B Oral Oncol 1995;31B(3):181–7.

15. Goldstein BY, Chang S-C, Hashibe M, et al. Alcohol consumption and cancers of the oral cavity and pharynx from 1988 to 2009: an update. Eur J Cancer Prev 2010;19(6):431–65.

16. Franceschi S, Levi F, Maso LD, et al. Cessation of alcohol drinking and risk of cancer of the oral cavity and pharynx. Int J Cancer 2000;85(6):787–90.

17. Dahlstrom KR, Little JA, Zafereo ME, et al. Squamous cell carcinoma of the head and neck in never smoker-never drinkers: a descriptive epidemiologic study. Head Neck 2008;30(1):75–84.

18. Wiseman SM, Swede H, Stoler DL, et al. Squamous Cell Carcinoma of the Head and Neck in Nonsmokers and Nondrinkers: An Analysis of Clinicopathologic Characteristics and Treatment Outcomes. Ann Surg Oncol 2003;10(5):551–7.

19. Patel SC, Carpenter WR, Tyree S, et al. Increasing incidence of oral tongue squamous cell carcinoma in young white women, age 18 to 44 years. J Clin Oncol 2011;29(11):1488–94.

20. Ng JH, Iyer NG, Tan M-H, et al. Changing epidemiology of oral squamous cell carcinoma of the tongue: A global study. Head & Neck 2017;39(2):297–304.

21. Mizuno K, Takeuchi M, Kikuchi M, et al. Outcomes in patients diagnosed with tongue cancer before and after the age of 45 years. Oral Oncol 2020;110: 105010.

22. Piemonte ED, Lazos JP, Brunotto M. Relationship between chronic trauma of the oral mucosa, oral potentially malignant disorders and oral cancer. J Oral Pathol Med 2010;39(7):513–7.

23. Vial T, Descotes J. Immunosuppressive drugs and cancer. Toxicology 2003; 185(3):229–40.

24. IARC Working Group on the Evaluation of Carcinogenic Risks to Humans. Betel-quid and areca-nut chewing and some areca-nut derived nitrosamines. IARC Monogr Eval Carcinog Risks Hum 2004;85:1–334.

25. Thomas SJ, Bain CJ, Battistutta D, et al. Betel quid not containing tobacco and oral cancer: A report on a case–control study in Papua New Guinea and a meta-analysis of current evidence. Int J Cancer 2007;120(6):1318–23.

26. Pan C, Issaeva N, Yarbrough WG. HPV-driven oropharyngeal cancer: current knowledge of molecular biology and mechanisms of carcinogenesis. Cancers of the Head & Neck 2018;3(1):12.
27. Amagasa T, Yamashiro M, Uzawa N. Oral premalignant lesions: from a clinical perspective. Int J Clin Oncol 2011;16(1):5–14.
28. Pinto AC, Caramês J, Francisco H, et al. Malignant transformation rate of oral leukoplakia-systematic review. Oral Surg Oral Med Oral Pathol Oral Radiol 2020;129(6):600–11.e2.
29. Shafer WG, Waldron CA. Erythroplakia of the oral cavity. Cancer 1975;36(3):1021–8.
30. Villa A, Villa C, Abati S. Oral cancer and oral erythroplakia: an update and implication for clinicians. Aust Dent J 2011;56(3):253–6.
31. Iocca O, Sollecito TP, Alawi F, et al. Potentially malignant disorders of the oral cavity and oral dysplasia: A systematic review and meta-analysis of malignant transformation rate by subtype. Head Neck 2020;42(3):539–55.
32. Dammann F, Horger M, Mueller-Berg M, et al. Rational Diagnosis of Squamous Cell Carcinoma of the Head and Neck Region: Comparative Evaluation of CT, MRI, and 18FDG PET. Am J Roentgenology 2005;184(4):1326–31.
33. Seitz O, Chambron-Pinho N, Middendorp M, et al. 18F-Fluorodeoxyglucose-PET/CT to evaluate tumor, nodal disease, and gross tumor volume of oropharyngeal and oral cavity cancer: comparison with MR imaging and validation with surgical specimen. Neuroradiology 2009;51(10):677–86.
34. Pentenero M, Cistaro A, Brusa M, et al. Accuracy of 18F-FDG-PET/CT for staging of oral squamous cell carcinoma. Head & Neck 2008;30(11):1488–96.
35. Sarrión Pérez MG, Bagán JV, Jiménez Y, et al. Utility of imaging techniques in the diagnosis of oral cancer. J Cranio-Maxillofacial Surg 2015;43(9):1880–94.
36. Xu G-Z, Guan D-J, He Z-Y. 18)FDG-PET/CT for detecting distant metastases and second primary cancers in patients with head and neck cancer. A meta-analysis. Oral Oncol 2011;47(7):560–5.
37. Tirelli G, Gatto A, Boscolo Nata F, et al. Prognosis of oral cancer: a comparison of the staging systems given in the 7th and 8th editions of the American Joint Committee on Cancer Staging Manual. Br J Oral Maxillofac Surg 2018;56(1):8–13.
38. Moeckelmann N, Ebrahimi A, Tou YK, et al. Prognostic implications of the 8th edition American Joint Committee on Cancer (AJCC) staging system in oral cavity squamous cell carcinoma. Oral Oncol 2018;85:82–6.
39. Pollaers K, Hinton-Bayre A, Friedland PL, et al. AJCC 8th Edition oral cavity squamous cell carcinoma staging - Is it an improvement on the AJCC 7th Edition? Oral Oncol 2018;82:23–8.
40. Spiro RH, Huvos AG, Wong GY, et al. Predictive value of tumor thickness in squamous carcinoma confined to the tongue and floor of the mouth. Am J Surg 1986;152(4):345–50.
41. Bundgaard T, Rossen K, Henriksen SD, et al. Histopathologic parameters in the evaluation of T1 squamous cell carcinomas of the oral cavity. Head Neck 2002;24(7):656–60.
42. Zanoni DK, Montero PH, Migliacci JC, et al. Survival outcomes after treatment of cancer of the oral caviTY (1985-2015). Oral Oncol 2019;90:115–21.
43. Oral Cancer 5-Year Survival Rates by Race, Gender, and Stage of Diagnosis | National Institute of Dental and Craniofacial Research. Available at: https://www.nidcr.nih.gov/research/data-statistics/oral-cancer/survival-rates. Accessed July 8, 2021.

44. Gil Z, Carlson DL, Boyle JO, et al. Lymph node density is a significant predictor of outcome in patients with oral cancer. Cancer 2009;115(24):5700–10.

45. National Comprehensive Cancer Network. Head and Neck Cancers (Version 3.2021). Available at: https://www.nccn.org/guidelines/guidelines-detail?category=1&id=1437. Accessed July 9, 2021.

46. Smith JE, Suh JD, Erman A, et al. Risk Factors Predicting Aspiration After Free Flap Reconstruction of Oral Cavity and Oropharyngeal Defects. Arch Otolaryngol Head Neck Surg 2008;134(11):1205.

47. Looser KG, Shah JP, Strong EW. The significance of "positive" margins in surgically resected epidermoid carcinomas. Head Neck Surg 1978;1(2):107–11.

48. Sutton DN, Brown JS, Rogers SN, et al. The prognostic implications of the surgical margin in oral squamous cell carcinoma. Int J Oral Maxillofac Surg 2003; 32(1):30–4.

49. Ganly I, Patel S, Shah J. Early stage squamous cell cancer of the oral tongue–clinicopathologic features affecting outcome. Cancer 2012;118(1):101–11.

50. Pathak KA, Nason RW, Penner C, et al. Impact of use of frozen section assessment of operative margins on survival in oral cancer. Oral Surg Oral Med Oral Pathol Oral Radiol Endod 2009;107(2):235–9.

51. Buchakjian MR, Tasche KK, Robinson RA, et al. Association of main specimen and tumor bed margin status with local recurrence and survival in oral cancer surgery. JAMA Otolaryngol Head Neck Surg 2016;142(12):1191–8.

52. Mair M, Nair D, Nair S, et al. Intraoperative gross examination vs frozen section for achievement of adequate margin in oral cancer surgery. Oral Surg Oral Med Oral Pathol Oral Radiol 2017;123(5):544–9.

53. Bulbul MG, Tarabichi O, Sethi RK, et al. Does clearance of positive margins improve local control in oral cavity cancer? a meta-analysis. Otolaryngol Head Neck Surg 2019;161(2):235–44.

54. Pfister DG, Spencer S, Adelstein D, et al. NCCN guidelines insights: head and neck cancers, version 3. J Natl Compr Canc Netw 2021. Available at: https://www.nccn.org/guidelines/guidelines-detail?category=1&id=1437. Accessed July 9, 2021.

55. Recommendations | Cancer of the upper aerodigestive tract: assessment and management in people aged 16 and over | Guidance | NICE. https://www.nice.org.uk/guidance/ng36/chapter/Recommendations#treatment-of-early-stage-disease. [Accessed 9 July 2021]. Accessed.

56. D'Cruz AK, Vaish R, Kapre N, et al. Elective versus therapeutic neck dissection in node-negative oral cancer. N Engl J Med 2015;373(6):521–9.

57. Hutchison IL, Ridout F, Cheung SMY, et al. Nationwide randomised trial evaluating elective neck dissection for early stage oral cancer (SEND study) with meta-analysis and concurrent real-world cohort. Br J Cancer 2019;121(10): 827–36.

58. Melchers LJ, Schuuring E, van Dijk BAC, et al. Tumour infiltration depth ≩4mm is an indication for an elective neck dissection in pT1cN0 oral squamous cell carcinoma. Oral Oncol 2012;48(4):337–42.

59. van Lanschot CGF, Klazen YP, de Ridder MAJ, et al. Depth of invasion in early stage oral cavity squamous cell carcinoma: The optimal cut-off value for elective neck dissection. Oral Oncol 2020;111:104940.

60. Scher ED, Romesser PB, Chen C, et al. Definitive chemoradiation for primary oral cavity carcinoma: A single institution experience. Oral Oncol 2015;51(7):709–15.

61. Spiotto MT, Jefferson G, Wenig B, et al. Differences in survival with surgery and postoperative radiotherapy compared with definitive chemoradiotherapy for oral

cavity cancer: a national cancer database analysis. JAMA Otolaryngology Head Neck Surg 2017;143(7):691–9.

62. Foster CC, Melotek JM, Brisson RJ, et al. Definitive chemoradiation for locally-advanced oral cavity cancer: A 20-year experience. Oral Oncol 2018;80:16–22.

63. Sasaki M, Aoki T, Karakida K, et al. Postoperative follow-up strategy in patients with oral squamous cell carcinoma. J Oral Maxillofac Surg 2011;69(6):e105–11.

64. Brands MT, Smeekens EAJ, Takes RP, et al. Time patterns of recurrence and second primary tumors in a large cohort of patients treated for oral cavity cancer. Cancer Med 2019;8(12):5810–9.

Management of Malignant Salivary Gland Conditions

John Pang, MD[a], Jeffrey J. Houlton, MD[b],*

KEYWORDS

- Salivary gland • Cancer • Carcinoma • Parotid • Submandibular

KEY POINTS

- Fine-needle aspiration is the preferred histologic diagnostic method in the workup of salivary masses.
- Surgery represents the mainstay of treatment of salivary cancers, followed by adjuvant radiation and/or chemotherapy for select cases.
- An aggressive parotid mass in a patient with a history of untreated/recurrent pleomorphic carcinoma is carcinoma ex pleomorphic adenoma until proved otherwise.
- A major tenant of salivary cancer resection is not to sacrifice facial nerve except in instances of gross encasement and inability to dissect tumor off of the nerve, as multiple studies have not found a survival advantage to nerve sacrifice.

BACKGROUND

Salivary malignancies represent a heterogeneous spectrum of pathologies with diverse features in presentation with evolving treatment paradigms. Such cancers occur more commonly in the major (parotid, submandibular, and sublingual) salivary glands than the minor salivary glands. The incidence is 1 per 100,000 people per year, and the mean age of diagnosis is 64 years.[1] Among head and neck cancers, salivary cancers represent 6.5% of all cancers.[2] Five-year relative survival rates by stage are 95%, 69%, and 44%, for local, regional, and distant disease, respectively.[1]

Among the major glands, malignancy is least likely in the parotid gland, with 15% to 32% of parotid tumors being malignant, followed by 41% to 45% of submandibular tumors and 70% to 90% of sublingual tumors.[3] Minor salivary glands, of which there are hundreds, are dispersed throughout the mucosa of the head and neck, including the palate, pharynx, and floor of mouth. Malignancy rates of minor salivary gland tumors range from 40% in the palate region up to 90% in the floor of mouth.[3,4] As a general rule of the thumb, the larger a salivary gland is (parotid, followed by

---

[a] University of Washington, 1959 Northeast Pacific Street, Seattle, WA 98195, USA;
[b] Otolaryngology–Head and Neck Surgery, University of Washington, 1959 Northeast Pacific Street, Seattle, WA 98195, USA
* Corresponding author.
E-mail address: jhoulton@uw.edu

Surg Clin N Am 102 (2022) 325–333
https://doi.org/10.1016/j.suc.2021.12.008
0039-6109/22/© 2022 Elsevier Inc. All rights reserved.

submandibular, then sublingual/minor salivary), the lower the malignancy risk is of neoplasms found in that gland. In general, parotid neoplasms have a 20% risk of malignancy, submandibular neoplasms 50%, and minor salivary neoplasms 60%. However, the overall frequency of neoplasms is associated with the size of the gland, with parotid neoplasms being most common, then submandibular neoplasms, and finally sublingual/minor salivary.

RELEVANT ANATOMY

The reader is referred to more comprehensive citations for a detailed discussion of salivary gland anatomy,[5] but briefly the paired parotid glands are situated in the parotid space bilaterally. This space is bound by the superficial layer of the deep cervical fascia that overlies the superficial lobe of the gland and contains the parotid gland, as well as the intraparotid facial nerve, external carotid artery, and retromandibular vein. The parotid space sits just posterior to the masseter muscle, and is bordered on its deep surface by the ramus of the mandible, its posterior surface by the external ear and sternocleidomastoid, and superiorly it abuts the zygomatic arch and infratemporal fossa. The 5 terminal branches of the facial nerve (temporal/frontal, zygomatic, buccal, marginal mandibular, and cervical) arise within the parotid gland, as the nerve divides into a superior and inferior trunk shortly after emanating from the stylomastoid foramen. The nerve branches traverse the gland and then run just deep to the superficial layer of true temporal fascia superiorly and in the superficial layer of deep cervical fascia inferiorly, which is one fascial layer deep to platysma. The facial nerve can be weakened or paralyzed by direct tumor extension or by surgical dissection/ligation.

Submandibular glands are situated within the submandibular space, which is bound superomedially by the digastric and mylohyoid muscles, laterally by the mandible, and inferiorly by the hyoid bone. Occupying this space are the paired submandibular glands, facial vessels, and submandibular lymph nodes. Just superior to the submandibular space is the sublingual space, which is bound by the mylohyoid laterally and superomedially by the geniohyoid/genioglossus and intrinsic tongue muscles.

Parotid cancers carry a risk of invasion to the main trunk of the facial nerve and any of its branches, whereas submandibular tumors typically pose a risk to only the marginal mandibular nerve and less commonly the hypoglossal nerve. Sublingual tumors may present with weakness of both lingual and hypoglossal nerves.

Workup and Management

A history and physical examination will typically yield a palpable mass of the head and neck region. For parotid masses, the infraauricular and preauricular regions are common. Rarely, isolated deep lobe tumors may not be noticeable in patients with significant soft tissue and may be identified incidentally through imaging (see JH MRI). Localized masses should be differentiated from diffuse parotid swelling and tenderness, as the latter is a distinguishing feature of infectious/inflammatory causes. Pain is present in up to 40% of malignancies, and enlarged cervical lymph nodes, facial nerve palsy, and overlying skin infiltration suggest malignancy.[6] A history of radiation or prior facial/scalp skin cancers suggests malignancy as well.

Submandibular cancers present with a palpable mass inferior to the mandibular body. The most common causes tend to be low grade, and as such paresis of the marginal mandibular nerve is possible but rarely encountered on presentation. Minor salivary gland cancers can present anywhere along the upper aerodigestive tract, including sinonasal mucosa, palate, and oropharynx, with associated symptoms being related to mass effect, less likely invasion of adjacent structures.

IMAGING

Ultrasound is a low-cost imaging modality that provides sufficient diagnostic information for most of the salivary masses, including malignant. When performed by the surgeon and subsequent fine-needle aspiration, diagnostic accuracy of ultrasound-guided fine-needle aspiration is greater than 90%.[7] In certain clinical scenarios, specifically when there is concern for location of a malignant lesion adjacent to or invading the facial nerve, additional axial imaging such as computed tomography with contrast or MRI is indicated. Specifically, MRI is especially helpful when evaluating salivary cancers to evaluate for facial nerve involvement in parotid cancers and perineural skull base involvement (trigeminal ganglion) in appropriate minor salivary tumors. Furthermore, deep lobe parotid tumors are often difficult to visualize fully on ultrasound alone, and characteristics of any parapharyngeal extension are often obscured in ultrasonography by the mandibular ramus. Diffusion-weighted imaging can identify with more accuracy involvement of the facial nerve and characterize the degree of involvement as likely extracranial only or including the vertical segment within the mastoid bone.[8] This information is vital to surgical planning when there is the potential for facial nerve sacrifice with or without subsequent nerve grafting.

Pathologic Diagnosis

Overwhelming evidence supports fine-needle aspiration as the first-line diagnostic method of choice for salivary masses.[9–11] Fine-needle aspiration, when negative for malignancy, is accurate in 90% to 95% of cases and when positive for malignancy, is accurate in 75% to 93% of cases.[12] In an effort to improve consistency of reporting for salivary gland specimens, in 2015 the Milan System was developed. Mirroring the Bethesda system for thyroid nodule reporting, the Milan system consists of 6 classifications across a spectrum of benign to malignant lesions.[13] Initial reports demonstrate potential to improve communication between pathologists and clinicians.[14]

The most common salivary gland cancer is mucoepidermoid carcinoma, which is commonly slow growing and low grade as opposed to aggressive and high grade. Adenoid cystic carcinoma develops often in minor salivary glands in the oral cavity, including palate, buccal space, and floor of mouth. This entity has a proclivity for perineural invasion and often causes pain and paralysis. Acinic cell carcinomas, although rare, emanate from salivary acini (saliva-producing cells) and are most commonly found in the parotid gland. Melanoma and squamous cell carcinomas of the head and neck also metastasize to the parotid gland as first or second echelon nodal basins. Metastatic cutaneous skin cancers commonly present as a parotid mass in elderly patients with a history of sun exposure. Because the list of possible pathologic entities is lengthy, the reader is directed toward additional excellent resources on this topic.[15,16] **Box 1** lists the World Health Organization Classification of Head and Neck Tumors, Salivary Gland, 4th edition.[17]

A definitive pathologic diagnosis can be achieved with core biopsy but is rarely necessary before proceeding with treatment. Core biopsy provides the pathologist with more tissue for analysis and achieves slightly higher sensitivity and specificity for diagnosis than fine-needle aspiration (94% and 98%, respectively as reported by Kim and colleagues).[18] However, the most of the surgeons proceed to surgery without a specific histologic diagnosis, as even the most common benign pathology (pleomorphic adenoma) poses an increased risk of neoplastic conversion to carcinoma ex pleomorphic adenoma over time. Therefore, the role of core biopsy is often limited in scenarios when surgery may be best avoided, such as differentiating a

---

Box 1
World Health Organization classification of salivary tumors, 4th edition

Malignant Tumors
  Mucoepidermoid carcinoma
  Adenoid cystic carcinoma
  Acinic cell carcinoma
  Polymorphous adenocarcinoma
  Clear cell carcinoma
  Basal cell adenocarcinoma
  Intraductal carcinoma
  Adenocarcinoma, not otherwise specified
  Salivary duct carcinoma
  Myoepithelial carcinoma
  Epithelial-myoepithelial carcinoma
  Carcinoma ex pleomorphic adenoma
  Secretory carcinoma
  Sebaceous adenocarcinoma
  Carcinosarcoma
  Poorly differentiated carcinoma
  Lymphoepithelial carcinoma
  Squamous cell carcinoma
  Oncocytic carcinoma
  Sialoblastoma

Benign Tumors
  Pleomorphic adenoma
  Myoepithelioma
  Basal cell adenoma
  Warthin tumor
  Oncocytoma
  Lymphadenoma
  Cystadenoma
  Sialadenoma papilliferum
  Ductal papillomas
  Sebaceous adenoma
  Canalicular adenoma and other ductal adenomas

Nonneoplastic Epithelial Lesions
  Sclerosing polycystic adenosis
  Nodular oncocytic hyperplasia
  Lymphoepithelial sialadenitis
  Intercalated duct hyperplasia

Benign Soft Tissue Lesions
  Hemangioma
  Lipoma/sialolipoma
  Nodular fasciitis
  Hematolymphoid tumors
  Extranodal marginal zone lymphoma of mucosa-associated lymphoid tissue (MALT lymphoma)

---

benign versus malignant process in an elderly patient wanting to forgo surgery. Core biopsy can also be helpful in cases where facial nerve sacrifice is being contemplated, especially in patients who present with no or limited signs of weakness, to clarify the surgical plan preoperatively. An alternative to preoperative core biopsy in these situations is to send intraoperative frozen tissue analysis of tumor invading facial nerve to justify sacrifice.

Staging and Prognosis

The TNM version 8 staging criteria by the American Joint Committee on Cancer classifies major salivary gland cancers from T1 to T4. T4 disease deserves further discussion for management purposes, as T4a is characterized by skin, mandible, ear canal, or facial nerve involvement.[19] While resec, composite resection is likely indicated, and the surgeon should be prepared to perform reconstruction as indicated, including regional/free flaps and reanimation procedures at the time of resection. T4b classification is characterized by skull base, pterygoid plate, and carotid artery encasement and in most scenarios is feasibly unresec without undue morbidity. Nodal disease ranges from N0 to N3b, with N3b disease reserved for clinical extranodal extension.

Salivary cancers typically have a favorable prognosis, especially when localized, as they are typically low grade. Surveillance, Epidemiology, and End Results Program data shows 95% 5-year relative survival for localized cancer, 69% for regional disease, and 44% for distant disease, with all stages combined being 75%.[20] For high-grade malignancies, patients with early stage disease (T1-2N0M0) have more than 90% 5-year disease-specific survival rates, but survival declines to 45% and 21% for nodal involvement and distant metastasis, respectively.[21]

SURGICAL TREATMENT

The first reported parotidectomy was by the German surgeon Lorenz Heister, and subsequently George McClellan performed the first parotidectomy for cancer in the United States, sacrificing facial nerve in performing total parotidectomy in 11/30 patients.[22] Surgery is the mainstay of treatment of salivary cancers, followed by adjuvant radiotherapy and chemotherapy in select cases. Rare exceptions to this pathway include aggressive cancers (ie, T4b disease) or cancers in elderly patients, in which case neoadjuvant chemotherapy or palliative treatment are acceptable alternatives. National Comprehensive Cancer Network guidelines recommend up front surgical therapy for all salivary tumors except T4b disease.

Identification of the facial nerve and its branches is critical in parotid surgery, as the surgeon should be familiar with important anatomic landmarks.[23] Identification and dissection of salivary cancers off of the facial nerve is often augmented with a facial nerve monitor. Although intraoperative facial nerve monitoring is certainly not ubiquitous, it is used by the overwhelming majority of surgeons. A recent systematic review and meta-analysis demonstrated a significant decrease in temporary and permanent weakness with intraoperative facial nerve monitoring (23% vs 38% and 6% vs 14%; $P = .001$).[24]

Adequacy of margin status is an ongoing topic of research. Wide soft tissue margins are often not feasible without undue morbidity due to proximity of the facial nerve. Moreover, prognosis hinges on histologic grade, perineural invasion, T classification, and nodal status in addition to margin status.[25] A major tenant of salivary cancer resection is not to sacrifice facial nerve except in instances of gross encasement and inability to dissect tumor off of the nerve, as multiple studies have not found a survival advantage to nerve sacrifice.[26–28] A recent retrospective review of 70 cases by Swendseid found that in 40/75 (53%) of patients with salivary cancer, facial nerve sparing was possible. Patients who required facial nerve sacrifice were those who presented with facial nerve weakness (100% sacrifice rate) or had preoperative pain (80%).

For low-grade tumors, most surgeons aim to achieve margins less than 1 cm. For high-grade tumors (high-grade mucoepidermoid carcinoma, salivary ductal carcinoma, squamous cell carcinoma, and carcinoma ex pleomorphic adenoma), Ord and colleagues recommend wider margins with postoperative radiation and elective neck dissection even in the clinically negative neck. Minor salivary glands most commonly involve the oral cavity, where obtaining negative margins not only requires modifications in technical planning but also reconstructive options including free tissue transfer. In these cases, the effect of a close or positive margin was studied by Hay and colleagues, who found hazard ratio of 1.56 for worse overall survival (confidence interval [CI] 95 1.02–2.39), which although significant, had a weaker effect than both stage and histology risk category (hazard ratio [HR] 4–6 and 1.3–2.4, respectively).

Role of Neck Dissection

Dissection of regional lymph nodes is standard of care when patients present with N+ disease (ie, clinically involved nodal disease). Of recent debate is when an elective neck dissection of an N0 neck without clinical nodal disease is indicated, as neck dissections do carry a low but definite risk of weakness to the marginal mandibular nerve, shoulder strength via spinal accessory, as well as hypoglossal and vagus nerves. Moreover, adjuvant radiation is recommended by National Comprehensive Cancer Network (NCCN) in completely resected adenoid cystic, intermediate or high-grade tumors, positive perineural invasion, positive lymphovascular invasion, close/positive margins, and T3/T4 tumors.[29]

Moss and colleagues performed a systematic review of elective neck dissection for mucoepidermoid carcinoma and found that occult nodal disease reaches 35% in patients with high-grade tumors, arguing for elective neck dissection in certain cases.[30] Harbison and colleagues analyzed data from National Cancer Database, in nearly 1600 patients with high-grade salivary cancers, and found no survival benefit to additional neck dissection in patients undergoing surgery followed by radiation.[31]

Adjuvant Radiation

Adjuvant radiation gives improved survival in patients with adverse pathologic features and is recommended by NCCN (see earlier discussion).[29] Radiation alone has even been reported to result in cure in 20% of salivary cancers.[32] A large retrospective cohort by Terhaard and colleagues found that postoperative radiation resulted in better 10-year local control significantly compared with surgery alone in T3 and T4 tumors (84% vs 18%), close margins (95% vs 55%), incomplete resection (82% vs 44), and perineural invasion (88% vs 60%).[33] In analyzing more than 8000 patients in the National Cancer Database, Bakst and colleagues found that adjuvant radiation conferred a significant survival advantage of HR 0.76 (CI 95 0.64–0.91) in patients with high-risk tumors, defined as extracapsular extension or positive margin). However, patients with T3/T4 disease, N+ disease, lymphovascular invasion, and adenoid cystic histology did not seem to benefit from adjuvant radiation (HR 1.01, CI 95 0.85–1.20).[34]

CONTROVERSIES AND FUTURE DIRECTIONS

Emerging evidence continues to influence several topics within salivary cancers. Notably, salivary duct carcinoma is the most aggressive of all salivary subtypes, although it presents rarely but often at advanced stages. Most of the patients survive less than 3 years.[35] Recent sequencing analysis of salivary duct carcinoma found the most frequent mutation to be in *TP53*.[36] Copy number gain of *ErbB2*, *EGFR* overexpression, androgen receptor overexpression, and alterations in PI3K/AKT/mTOR pathway have also been reported.[36] Trastuzumab, an inhibitor of ErbB2/HER-2, in particular has shown promise with severale complete responses on trastuzumab maintenance therapy. More than half of the patients in a small case series of maintenance trastuzumab have had durable responses, suggesting promise in targeted therapy for this aggressive histology.[37,38]

CLINICS CARE POINTS

- Five-year relative survival rates by stage are 95%, 69%, and 44%, for local, regional, and distant disease, respectively.
- Fine-needle aspiration, when negative for malignancy, is accurate in 90% to 95% of cases and when positive for malignancy, is accurate in 75% to 93% of cases.
- A major tenant of salivary cancer resection is not to sacrifice facial nerve except in instances of gross encasement and inability to dissect tumor off of the nerve, as multiple studies have not found a survival advantage to nerve sacrifice.
- Adjuvant radiation is recommended by NCCN in completely resected adenoid cystic, intermediate- or high-grade tumors, positive perineural invasion, positive lymphovascular invasion, close/positive margins, and T3/T4 tumors.

DISCLOSURE

The authors have nothing to disclose.

REFERENCES

1. American Cancer Society. Salivary gland cancer. Available at: https://www.cancer.org/cancer/salivary-gland-cancer/. Accessed May 31, 2021.
2. Carvalho AL, Nishimoto IN, Califano JA, et al. Trends in incidence and prognosis for head and neck cancer in the United States: a site-specific analysis of the SEER database. Int J Cancer 2005;114(5):806–16. https://doi.org/10.1002/ijc.20740.
3. Guzzo M, Locati LD, Prott FJ, et al. Major and minor salivary gland tumors. Crit Rev Oncol Hematol 2010;74(2):134–48. https://doi.org/10.1016/j.critrevonc.2009.10.004.
4. Waldron CA, el-Mofty SK, Gnepp DR. Tumors of the intraoral minor salivary glands: a demographic and histologic study of 426 cases. Oral Surg Oral Med Oral Pathol 1988;66(3):323–33. https://doi.org/10.1016/0030-4220(88)90240-x.
5. Witt R. Surgery of the salivary glands. Switzerland: Springer; 2020.
6. Stodulski D, Mikaszewski B, Stankiewicz C. Signs and symptoms of parotid gland carcinoma and their prognostic value. Int J Oral Maxillofac Surg 2012;41(7): 801–6. https://doi.org/10.1016/j.ijom.2011.12.020.
7. Lanišnik B, Levart P, Čizmarevič B, et al. Surgeon-performed ultrasound with fine-needle aspiration biopsy for the diagnosis of parotid gland tumors. Head Neck 2021;43(6):1739–46. https://doi.org/10.1002/hed.26630.
8. El Kininy W, Roddy D, Davy S, et al. Magnetic resonance diffusion weighted imaging using constrained spherical deconvolution-based tractography of the extracranial course of the facial nerve. Oral Surg Oral Med Oral Pathol Oral Radiol 2020;130(2):e44–56. https://doi.org/10.1016/j.oooo.2019.12.012.
9. Boldes T, Hilly O, Alkan U, et al. Accuracy, predictability and prognostic implications of fine-needle aspiration biopsy for parotid gland tumours: a retrospective case series. Clin Otolaryngol 2021. https://doi.org/10.1111/coa.13795.
10. Reerds STH, Van Engen-Van Grunsven ACH, van den Hoogen FJA, et al. Accuracy of parotid gland FNA cytology and reliability of the Milan System for

reporting salivary gland cytopathology in clinical practice. Cancer Cytopathol 2021. https://doi.org/10.1002/cncy.22435.

11. Stewart CJ, MacKenzie K, McGarry GW, et al. Fine-needle aspiration cytology of salivary gland: a review of 341 cases. Diagn Cytopathol 2000;22(3):139–46. https://doi.org/10.1002/(sici)1097-0339(20000301)22:3<139::aid-dc2>3.0.co; 2-a.

12. Feinstein AJ, Alonso J, Yang SE, et al. Diagnostic accuracy of fine-needle aspiration for parotid and submandibular gland lesions. Otolaryngology–head neck Surg 2016;155(3):431–6. https://doi.org/10.1177/0194599816643041.

13. Pusztaszeri M, Rossi ED, Baloch ZW, et al. Salivary gland fine needle aspiration and introduction of the milan reporting system. Adv Anat Pathol 2019;26(2): 84–92. https://doi.org/10.1097/pap.0000000000000224.

14. Mullen D, Gibbons D. A retrospective comparison of salivary gland fine needle aspiration reporting with the Milan system for reporting salivary gland cytology. Cytopathology 2020;31(3):208–14. https://doi.org/10.1111/cyt.12811.

15. Carlson ER, Schlieve T. Salivary gland malignancies. Oral Maxillofac Surg Clin North Am 2019;31(1):125–44. https://doi.org/10.1016/j.coms.2018.08.007.

16. Zarbo RJ. Salivary gland neoplasia: a review for the practicing pathologist. Mod Pathol 2002;15(3):298–323. https://doi.org/10.1038/modpathol.3880525.

17. El-Naggar AK, Chan JKC, Rubin Grandis J, et al, International Agency for Research on C. WHO classification of head and neck tumours. 2017.

18. Kim HJ, Kim JS. Ultrasound-guided core needle biopsy in salivary glands: a meta-analysis. Laryngoscope 2018;128(1):118–25. https://doi.org/10.1002/lary. 26764.

19. Amin MB, Edge S, Greene F, et al, editors. AJCC cancer staging manual. 8th edition. Springer International Publishing: American Joint Commission on Cancer; 2017.

20. Survival rates for salivary gland cancer. Available at: https://www.cancer.org/ cancer/salivary-gland-cancer/detection-diagnosis-staging/survival-rates.html.

21. Jang JY, Choi N, Ko YH, et al. Treatment outcomes in metastatic and localized high-grade salivary gland cancer: high chance of cure with surgery and post-operative radiation in T1-2 N0 high-grade salivary gland cancer. BMC Cancer 2018;18(1):672. https://doi.org/10.1186/s12885-018-4578-0.

22. Melo GM, Cervantes O, Abrahao M, et al. A brief history of salivary gland surgery. Rev Col Bras Cir 2017;44(4):403–12. https://doi.org/10.1590/0100-69912017004004. Uma breve história da cirurgia das glândulas salivares.

23. Kochhar A, Larian B, Azizzadeh B. Facial nerve and parotid gland anatomy. Otolaryngol Clin North Am 2016;49(2):273–84. https://doi.org/10.1016/j.otc.2015. 10.002.

24. Chiesa-Estomba CM, Larruscain-Sarasola E, Lechien JR, et al. Facial nerve monitoring during parotid gland surgery: a systematic review and meta-analysis. Eur Arch Otorhinolaryngol 2021;278(4):933–43. https://doi.org/10.1007/s00405-020-06188-0.

25. Ord RA, Ghazali N. Margin analysis: malignant salivary gland neoplasms of the head and neck. Oral Maxillofac Surg Clin North Am 2017;29(3):315–24. https:// doi.org/10.1016/j.coms.2017.03.008.

26. Terhaard C, Lubsen H, Tan B, et al. Facial nerve function in carcinoma of the parotid gland. Eur J Cancer 2006;42(16):2744–50. https://doi.org/10.1016/j.ejca. 2006.06.010.

27. Terakedis BE, Hunt JP, Buchmann LO, et al. The prognostic significance of facial nerve involvement in carcinomas of the parotid gland. Am J Clin Oncol 2017; 40(3):323–8. https://doi.org/10.1097/coc.0000000000000157.
28. Guntinas-Lichius O, Klussmann JP, Schroeder U, et al. Primary parotid malignoma surgery in patients with normal preoperative facial nerve function: outcome and long-term postoperative facial nerve function. Laryngoscope 2004;114(5):949–56. https://doi.org/10.1097/00005537-200405000-00032.
29. National Comprehensive Cancer Network. Clinical Practice Guidelines in Oncology. Version 1.2020. Available at: https://www.nccn.org/professionals/physician_gls/pdf/head-and-neck.pdf. Accessed May 8, 2020.
30. Moss WJ, Coffey CS, Brumund KT, et al. What is the role of elective neck dissection in low-, intermediate-, and high-grade mucoepidermoid carcinoma? Laryngoscope 2016;126(1):11–3. https://doi.org/10.1002/lary.25588.
31. Harbison RA, Gray AJ, Westling T, et al. The role of elective neck dissection in high-grade parotid malignancy: a hospital-based cohort study. Laryngoscope 2020;130(6):1487–95. https://doi.org/10.1002/lary.28238.
32. Mendenhall WM, Morris CG, Amdur RJ, et al. Radiotherapy alone or combined with surgery for salivary gland carcinoma. Cancer 2005;103(12):2544–50. https://doi.org/10.1002/cncr.21083.
33. Terhaard CH, Lubsen H, Rasch CR, et al. The role of radiotherapy in the treatment of malignant salivary gland tumors. Int J Radiat Oncol Biol Phys 2005;61(1): 103–11. https://doi.org/10.1016/j.ijrobp.2004.03.018.
34. Bakst RL, Su W, Ozbek U, et al. Adjuvant radiation for salivary gland malignancies is associated with improved survival: a National Cancer Database analysis. Adv Radiat Oncol 2017;2(2):159–66. https://doi.org/10.1016/j.adro.2017.03.008.
35. Schmitt NC, Kang H, Sharma A. Salivary duct carcinoma: an aggressive salivary gland malignancy with opportunities for targeted therapy. Oral Oncol 2017;74: 40–8. https://doi.org/10.1016/j.oraloncology.2017.09.008.
36. Chiosea SI, Williams L, Griffith CC, et al. Molecular characterization of apocrine salivary duct carcinoma. Am J Surg Pathol 2015;39(6):744–52. https://doi.org/10.1097/pas.0000000000000410.
37. Thorpe LM, Schrock AB, Erlich RL, et al. Significant and durable clinical benefit from trastuzumab in 2 patients with HER2-amplified salivary gland cancer and a review of the literature. Head & neck 2017;39(3):E40–4. https://doi.org/10.1002/hed.24634.
38. Shin DS, Sherry T, Kallen ME, et al. Human epidermal growth factor receptor 2 (HER-2/neu)-directed therapy for rare metastatic epithelial tumors with HER-2 amplification. Case Rep Oncol 2016;9(2):298–304. https://doi.org/10.1159/000445827.

Moving?

Make sure your subscription moves with you!

To notify us of your new address, find your **Clinics Account Number** (located on your mailing label above your name), and contact customer service at:

Email: journalscustomerservice-usa@elsevier.com

800-654-2452 (subscribers in the U.S. & Canada)
314-447-8871 (subscribers outside of the U.S. & Canada)

Fax number: 314-447-8029

Elsevier Health Sciences Division
Subscription Customer Service
3251 Riverport Lane
Maryland Heights, MO 63043

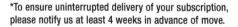

Printed and bound by CPI Group (UK) Ltd, Croydon, CR0 4YY

03/10/2024

01040483-0014